DIAGNOSTIC ULTRASOUND

Imaging and Blood Flow Measurements

SECOND EDITION

DIAGNOSTIC ULTRASOUND

Imaging and Blood Flow Measurements

SECOND EDITION

K. Kirk Shung

University of Southern California
Los Angeles, USA

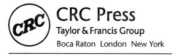

CRC Press
Taylor & Francis Group
Boca Raton London New York

CRC Press is an imprint of the
Taylor & Francis Group, an **informa** business

CRC Press
Taylor & Francis Group
6000 Broken Sound Parkway NW, Suite 300
Boca Raton, FL 33487-2742

First issued in paperback 2017

ISBN-13: 978-1-4665-8264-4 (hbk)
ISBN-13: 978-1-138-89288-0 (pbk)

Library of Congress Cataloging-in-Publication Data

Shung, K. Kirk, author.
    Diagnostic ultrasound : imaging and blood flow measurements / Kirk Shung. -- Second edition.
    p. ; cm.
    Includes bibliographical references.
    Summary: "This is a substantial revision of a respected work that details the latest advances in ultrasound technology related to biomedical applications. This includes such topics as elastography, portable scanners, ultrasound molecular imaging, preclinical high frequency imaging, 2D array and 4D imaging techniques. Each chapter has been considerably updated and expanded. A new chapter has been added on new developments such as elastography and minature scanners. New case studies and examples throughout the book are also included in this new edition"--Provided by publisher.
    ISBN 978-1-4665-8264-4 (hardback)
    I. Title.
    [DNLM: 1. Ultrasonography. 2. Laser-Doppler Flowmetry. 3. Ultrasonography, Doppler, Color--methods. WN 208]

    RC78.7.U4
    616.07'543--dc23   2014043870

Visit the Taylor & Francis Web site at
http://www.taylorandfrancis.com

and the CRC Press Web site at
http://www.crcpress.com

Dedication

This book is dedicated to my wife,
Linda, and three children,
Albert, Simon, and May, and their spouses,
Rini, Jenny, and Chris.

Contents

Preface

The field of medical imaging is advancing at a rapid pace. Imaging modalities such as x-ray radiography, x-ray computed tomography (CT), ultrasound, nuclear imaging, magnetic resonance imaging (MRI), and optical imaging have been used in biology and medicine to visualize anatomical structures as large as the lung and liver and as small as molecules. Ultrasound is considered the most cost-effective among them all. It is used routinely in hospitals and clinics for diagnosing a variety of diseases and is considered the tool of choice in obstetrics and cardiology because it is safe and capable of providing images in real time. New applications in preclinical or small animal imaging and cellular imaging are being explored.

Although there have been many clinical books published for ultrasound, very few technical books are available. Over the past 35 years, this has been a major problem for the author in teaching a graduate course in ultrasonic imaging at the Department of Bioengineering, Pennsylvania State University, and the Department of Biomedical Engineering, University of Southern California. It is for this purpose that this book was written. The book is intended to be a textbook for a senior-level or first-year graduate-level course in ultrasonic imaging in a biomedical engineering, electrical engineering, medical physics, or radiological sciences curriculum. An attempt has been made to minimize mathematical derivation and to place more emphasis on physical concepts. In this edition, several chapters, including the chapter on transducers, were greatly expanded. Chapter 1 gives an overview of the field of ultrasonic imaging and its role in diagnostic medicine relative to other imaging modalities. Chapters 2 and 3 describe the fundamental physics involved and a crucial device in ultrasound, ultrasonic transducers, respectively. Conventional imaging approaches and Doppler measurements are given in Chapters 4 and 5. More recent developments, including contrast imaging and 4D imaging, are described in Chapters 6 to 9. In Chapter 10, current status and standards on ultrasound bioeffects are reviewed. Chapter 11 discusses methods that have been used to measure ultrasonic properties of tissues. This chapter is optional and may be eliminated at the discretion of the instructor. At the end of each chapter a list of relevant references and further reading materials is given.

Material contained in the book should be more than sufficient for a one-semester graduate- or senior-level course.

The book should also be of interest to radiologists with some technical background and practicing engineers and physicists working in the imaging industry.

Acknowledgments

The author gratefully acknowledges the financial support provided by NIH grant #P41-T-R002182 during the period in which this book was written.

About the Author

K. Kirk Shung obtained a Ph.D. in electrical engineering from University of Washington, Seattle, in 1975. He is a Dean's Professor in Biomedical Engineering, an endowed position, at University of Southern California and has been the director of NIH Resource Center on Medical Ultrasonic Transducer Technology since 1997.

Dr. Shung is a life fellow of IEEE and a fellow of the Acoustical Society of America and American Institute of Ultrasound in Medicine. He is a founding fellow of American Institute of Medical and Biological Engineering. Dr. Shung received the IEEE Engineering in Medicine and Biology Society Early Career Award in 1985 and was the coauthor of a paper that received the best paper award for *IEEE Transactions on Ultrasonics, Ferroelectrics and Frequency Control* (UFFC) in 2000. He was selected as the distinguished lecturer for the IEEE UFFC society for 2002-2003. In 2010 and 2011, he received the Holmes Pioneer Award in Basic Science from American Institute of Ultrasound in Medicine and the academic career achievement award from the IEEE Engineering in Medicine and Biology Society.

Dr. Shung has published more than 500 papers and book chapters. He is the author of a textbook *Principles of Medical Imaging* published by Academic Press in 1992 and a textbook *Diagnostic Ultrasound: Imaging and Blood Flow Measurements* published by CRC press in 2005. He co-edited a book *Ultrasonic Scattering by Biological Tissues* published by CRC Press in 1993. Dr. Shung is currently serving as an associate editor of *IEEE Transactions on Ultrasonics, Ferroelectrics and Frequency Control*, *IEEE Transactions on Biomedical and Engineering*, and *Medical Physics*. Dr. Shung's research interest is in ultrasonic transducers, high frequency ultrasonic imaging, ultrasound microbeam, and ultrasonic scattering in tissues.

chapter one

Introduction

1.1 History

The potential of ultrasound as an imaging modality was realized as early as the late 1940s, when several groups of investigators around the world utilizing sonar and radar technology developed during World War II started exploring medical diagnostic capabilities of ultrasound (Goldberg and Kimmelman, 1988). John Wild and John Reid in Minnesota developed a prototype B-mode ultrasonic imaging instrument and were able to demonstrate the capability of ultrasound for imaging and characterization of cancerous tissues in the early 1950s at frequencies as high as 15 MHz. John Wild's pioneering effort and accomplishment were recognized with the Japan prize in 1991. At the same time, Douglas Howry and Joseph Holms at the University of Colorado at Denver, apparently unaware of the effort by Wild and Reid, also built an ultrasonic imaging device with which they produced cross-sectional images of the arm and leg. In Japan, starting in the late 1940s, medical applications of ultrasound were explored by Kenji Tanaka and Toshio Wagai. Two Japanese investigators, Drs. Shigeo Satomura and Yasuhara Nimura, were credited for the earliest development of ultrasonic Doppler devices for monitoring tissue motion and blood flow in 1955. Virtually simultaneously with the work going on in Japan and in the United States, Drs. Inge Edler and Hellmuth Hertz at the University of Lund in Sweden worked on echocardiography, an ultrasound imaging technique for imaging cardiac structures and monitoring cardiac functions. In parallel with these developments in the diagnostic front, William Fry and his colleagues at the University of Illinois at Urbana worked on using a high-intensity ultrasound beam to treat neurological disorders in the brain. The primary form of ultrasonic imaging to date has been that of a pulse-echo mode. The principle is very similar to that of sonar and radar. In essence, following an ultrasonic pulse transmission, echoes from the medium being interrogated are detected and used to form an image. Many terminologies used in ultrasound are imported from the field of sonar and radar. Although pulse-echo ultrasound had been used since the 1950s to diagnose a variety of medical problems, it did not become a widely accepted diagnostic tool until the early 1970s, when gray-scale ultrasound with nonlinear echo amplitude to gray-level mapping was introduced. Continuous-wave (CW) and pulsed-wave (PW) Doppler ultrasound devices for measuring blood flow also became available during that time. Duplex ultrasound scanners that combined both functions, allowing the imaging of anatomy and the measurement of blood flow with one single instrument, soon followed. Today, ultrasound is the second most utilized diagnostic imaging modality in medicine (second only to conventional x-ray) and is a critically important diagnostic tool of any medical facility.

Although ultrasound has been in existence for more than 40 years and is considered a mature technology by many, the field is by no means in a stagnant state. Technical advances are constantly being made. The introduction of contrast agents, harmonic imaging, flow and tissue displacement imaging, multidimensional imaging, and high-frequency imaging are just a few examples. In this book, these new developments, along with fundamental physics, instrumentation, system architecture, biological effects of ultrasound, and clinical applications, will be discussed in detail.

1.2 Role of ultrasound in medical imaging

Ultrasound not only complements the more traditional approaches such as x-ray, but also possesses unique characteristics that are advantageous in comparison to other competing modalities, such as x-ray computed tomography (CT), radionuclide emission tomography, and magnetic resonance imaging (MRI). More specifically, ultrasound (1) is a form of nonionizing radiation and is considered safe to the best of present knowledge, (2) is less expensive than imaging modalities of similar capabilities, (3) produces images in real time, unattainable at the present time by any other methods, (4) has a resolution in the millimeter range for the frequencies being clinically used today, which may be made better if the frequency is increased, (5) can yield blood flow information by applying the Doppler principle, and (6) is portable and thus can be easily transported to the bedside of a patient.

Ultrasound also has several drawbacks. Chief among them are that (1) bony structures and organs containing gases cannot be adequately imaged without introducing specialized procedures, (2) only a limited window is available for ultrasonic examination of certain organs such as the heart and neonatal brain, (3) it is operator skill dependent, and (4) it is sometimes impossible to obtain good images from certain types of patients, including obese patients.

The many advantages that ultrasound is capable of offering have allowed it to become a valuable diagnostic tool in such medical disciplines as cardiology, obstetrics, gynecology, surgery, pediatrics, radiology, and neurology, to name just a few. The relationship among ultrasound and other imaging modalities is a dynamic one. Ultrasound is the tool of choice in obstetrics primarily because of its noninvasive nature, its cost-effectiveness, and its real-time imaging capability. This role will not change in the foreseeable future. Ultrasound also enjoys similar success in cardiology, demonstrated by the fact that echocardiography is a training that every cardiologist must have. The future of ultrasound in cardiology, however, is not as rosy as in obstetrics because while ultrasound is progressing at a rapid rate, other competing imaging modalities, such as multislice spiral CT and MR, are also making great strides in improving the image acquisition rate and image quality. Ultrasound may lose ground in certain areas, but it may gain in other areas. Ultrasound mammography is an example of gradually gaining importance in breast cancer imaging. Nevertheless, at a time of heightened public concern with health care costs, the cost-effectiveness of an imaging tool is a crucial factor in planning diagnostic strategies. Diagnostic ultrasound is particularly attractive in this respect and is likely to remain a major diagnostic modality for many years to come.

Although the pace of development in therapeutic ultrasound has not been as striking as diagnostic ultrasound, significant progress has also been made in the past decades. These efforts have been primarily focused on developing better devices for hyperthermia, frequently in combination with chemotherapy or radiotherapy, for the treatment of tumors, and for high-intensity focused tissue ablation.

1.3 Purpose of the book

This book is written based upon the notes for a graduate course on ultrasound imaging that the author has been teaching at the Department of Bioengineering, Pennsylvania State University, and the Department of Biomedical Engineering, University of Southern California, since 1979. In the 2nd edition several chapters are expanded and updated. The book is intended to be a textbook for a senior- to graduate-level course in ultrasonic imaging. It should also be useful for physicists, engineers, clinicians, and sonographers who are interested in learning more about the technical side of diagnostic ultrasound as a reference.

References and Further Reading Materials

Cho ZH, Jones JP, and Singh M. *Foundations of medical imaging.* New York: John Wiley, 1993.
Christensen DA. *Ultrasonic bioinstrumentation.* New York: John Wiley, 1988.
Cobbold RSC. *Foundations of biomedical ultrasound.* Oxford: Oxford Press, 2007.
Evans DH and McDicken WN. *Doppler ultrasound: Physics, instrumentation, and signal processing.* 2nd ed. New York: John Wiley, 2000.
Goldberg BB and Kimmelman BA. *Medical diagnostic ultrasound: A retrospective on its 40th anniversary.* Laurel, MD: AIUM, 1988.

Jensen JA. *Estimation of blood velocities using ultrasound.* Cambridge: Cambridge University Press, 1996.

Kino GS. *Acoustic waves: Devices, imaging, and analog signal processing.* Englewood Cliffs, NJ: Prentice-Hall, 1987.

Kremkau FW. *Sonography: Principles and instruments.* 8th ed. St. Louis, MO: Saunders, 2010.

Shung KK, Smith MB, and Tsui BWN. *Principles of medical imaging.* San Diego: Academic Press, 1992.

Smith NB and Webb A. *Introduction to medical imaging: Physics, engineering, and clinical applications.* New York: Cambridge Press, 2010.

Suetens P. *Fundamentals of medical imaging.* Cambridge: Cambridge University Press, 2002.

Szabo TL. *Diagnostic ultrasound imaging: Inside out.* 2nd ed. Amsterdam: Elsevier Press, 2014.

Webb A. *Introduction to biomedical imaging.* Hoboken, NJ: Wiley, 2003.

Zagzebski JA. *Essentials of ultrasound physics.* St. Louis, MO: Mosby, 1996.

chapter two

Fundamentals of acoustic propagation

Ultrasound is a sound wave characterized by such parameters as pressure, particle (or medium) velocity, particle displacement, density, and temperature. It differs from other sound waves in that its frequency is higher than 20×10^3 cycles/s or 20 kilohertz (kHz). The audible range of the human ear is from 20 Hz to 20 kHz. Since ultrasound is a wave, it transmits energy just like an electromagnetic wave or radiation. Unlike an electromagnetic wave, however, sound requires a medium in which to travel, and thus cannot propagate in a vacuum. To better visualize how the sound propagates through a homogeneous medium, the medium can be modeled as a three-dimensional (3D) matrix of elements that may represent molecules, atoms, or elemental volumes or particles, separated by perfect elastic springs representing interelement forces. To simplify the matter even more, only a 2D lattice is shown in Figure 2.1, where the elements are represented by spheres. When a particle is pushed to a distance from its neutral position, the disturbance or force is transmitted to the adjacent particle by the spring. This creates a chain reaction. If the driving force is oscillating back and forth or in a sinusoidal manner, the particles respond by oscillating in the same way. The distance, U, traveled by the particle in the acoustic propagation is called particle or medium displacement, usually in the order of a few tenths of a nanometer in water. The velocity of the particle oscillating back and forth is called particle or medium velocity, u, and is in the order of a few centimeters per second in water. It must be noted that this velocity is different from the rate at which the energy is propagating through the medium. The velocity at which the ultrasound energy propagates through the medium is defined as the phase velocity or the sound propagation velocity, c. In water, $c \approx 1500$ m/s. This is illustrated in Figure 2.1, which shows that the sound velocity is much faster than the particle velocity. While the particle has only moved a short distance, the perturbation has already been transmitted to other particles over a much longer distance, U'. As a sinusoidal disturbance is propagated into a liquid medium, regions of medium compression and rarefaction are produced, as shown in Figure 2.2. If the pressure is plotted, it represents pressure variation over static ambient pressure. In air, the ambient pressure is 1 atm. In a water tank or in the human body, the

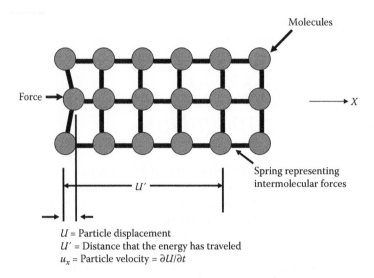

U = Particle displacement
U' = Distance that the energy has traveled
u_x = Particle velocity = $\partial U/\partial t$

Figure 2.1 A 2D matrix of molecules perturbed by an external force. The actual physical displacement of the lattices, U, is much smaller than the distance that the energy has traveled, represented by U'.

ambient pressure can be much higher than 1 atm. The displacement of the particles U is in the same direction as the direction of wave propagation X. This type of wave is called a longitudinal or compressional wave. The particle displacement in the rarefaction region is the largest, while it is the smallest in the compression. If the displacement of a particle versus distance or the displacement of a particle versus time is plotted, it can be seen that the particle moves in a sinusoidal format, as shown in Figure 2.3. The wavelength of a sound wave λ is defined as the distance between two points of the same phase in space, e.g., two peaks, or the distance for one

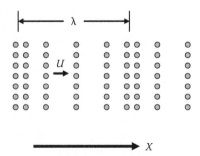

Figure 2.2 Regions of compression and rarefaction are formed in medium during sinusoidal wave propagation.

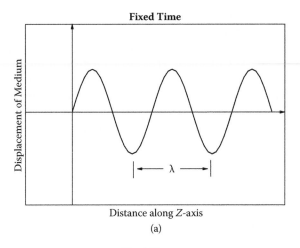

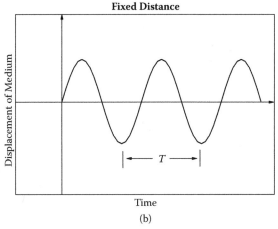

Figure 2.3 At a fixed time (a), the distance between two troughs or two peaks is defined as the wavelength, whereas at a fixed distance (b) the time lapse between two troughs is called the period.

cycle of wave to occur, at a fixed time, and the period, T, is defined as the time lapse between two points in time of the same phase, e.g., two peaks, or the time that it takes for one cycle of wave to occur at a fixed point in space. It follows from these definitions that

$$Tc = \lambda \tag{2.1}$$

Since frequency f is defined as $f = 1/T$, Equation (2.1) can be rewritten as

$$f\lambda = c \tag{2.2}$$

For an ultrasonic wave at 5 MHz, the wavelength is about 300 μm. It will be shown later that the spatial resolution of an ultrasonic imaging system, that is, its capability to spatially resolve an object, is primarily determined by the wavelength. The ultimate resolution that a 5 MHz ultrasonic imaging system can achieve is 300 μm. To improve the resolution, one option is to increase the frequency. In contrast, the wavelengths involved in x-ray or optical imaging are much shorter. Thus, for these modalities the frequency in general is not as critical when spatial resolution is concerned.

2.1 Stress and strain relationship

Acoustic propagation involves the propagation of a mechanical disturbance whose behavior can be derived from the fundamental concepts of strain and stress. An incremental cube of material within a body with external forces being applied to it is shown in Figure 2.4. The stress is defined as the tensile force exerted on the incremental cube by other parts of the body per unit area. On a unit surface perpendicular to the Z-axis or Z-plane, the stress can be separated into three components:

κ_{zz} = longitudinal stress in the Z-direction
κ_{yz} = shear stress in the Y-direction
κ_{xz} = shear stress in the X-direction

Similarly, κ_{zy}, κ_{yy}, κ_{xy} and κ_{zx}, κ_{yx}, κ_{xx} denote the stresses acted on in the Y- and X-planes. The deformation of the cube caused by an external force

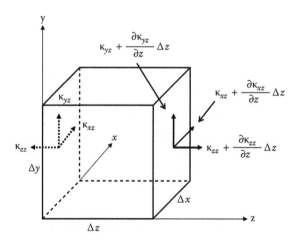

Figure 2.4 A stress is applied to a unit cube.

is described by the parameter strain, defined as the displacement per unit distance. The longitudinal strain in the Z-direction by the Z-plane is

$$\varepsilon_{zz} = \frac{\partial W}{\partial z}$$

and the shear strain in the X-direction by the Z-plane along the Z-axis is

$$\varepsilon_{xz} = \frac{\partial U}{\partial z}$$

where U, V, and W denote, respectively, the displacements in the X-, Y-, and Z-directions. They are functions of (x, y, z). The longitudinal and shear strains are graphically illustrated in Figure 2.5.

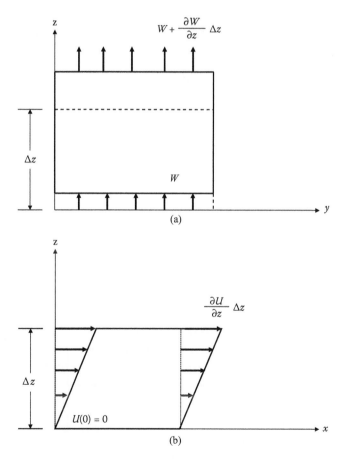

Figure 2.5 (a) Longitudinal strain of a Z-plane in the Z-direction. (b) Shear strain of a Z-plane in the Y-direction.

Under the condition of small displacements, the stress-strain relationships are linear (Malecki, 1969):

$$\kappa_{zz} = (v + 2\mu)\frac{\partial W}{\partial z} = (v + 2\mu)\varepsilon_{zz} \tag{2.3}$$

$$\kappa_{yz} = \mu\frac{\partial V}{\partial z} = \mu\varepsilon_{yz} \tag{2.4}$$

$$\kappa_{xz} = \mu\frac{\partial U}{\partial z} = \mu\varepsilon_{xz} \tag{2.5}$$

where v and μ are Lamé constants and μ is called the shear modulus because it relates the shear strain to the shear stress. The Lamé constants are related to the more conventional material constants, such as Young's modulus (E), bulk modulus (B), and Poisson's ratio (v_p), by the following equations:

$$E = \frac{\mu(3v + 2\mu)}{v + \mu}$$

$$B = v + \frac{2\mu}{3}$$

$$v_p = \frac{v}{2(v + \mu)}$$

The definitions of these conventional elastic constants can be better understood by examining Figure 2.6, where a square bar is shown under tensile stress. The Young's modulus is defined as the ratio of stress/strain or $\kappa_{zz}/\varepsilon_{zz}$, and the Poisson ratio is defined as the negative of the

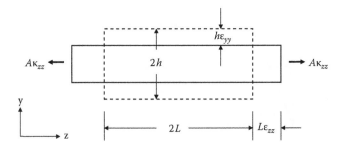

Figure 2.6 A bar of square cross section under tensile stress. $2L$ and A are, respectively, the length and cross-sectional A of the bar. $2h$ is the height.

ratio of strain in the transverse direction to the strain in the longitudinal direction, or $-\varepsilon_{yy}/\varepsilon_{zz}$.

The bulk modulus is the inverse of the compressibility of the medium. The compressibility (G) of a medium is defined as the negative of the change in volume per unit volume per unit change in pressure:

$$G = -\frac{1}{V}\frac{\partial V}{\partial p}$$

where V denotes the volume of a medium and p is pressure. Pressure is the normal compressional force applied on a surface per unit area of the surface and has a unit pascal or newton/m^2. Therefore, the pressure applied on a surface equals the negative of the stress applied on that surface. For a surface perpendicular to the Z-axis, $p = -\kappa_{zz}$. In a fluid where μ approaches 0, $B \sim v$ and $E \sim 0$.

2.2 Acoustic wave equation

The equation of motion in the Z-direction for an incremental cube, as shown in Figure 2.4, can be readily obtained by applying Newton's second law, that is, summing the net force applied on the cube in the Z-direction:

$$\frac{\partial \kappa_{zz}}{\partial z} + \frac{\partial \kappa_{zy}}{\partial y} + \frac{\partial \kappa_{zx}}{\partial x} = \rho\frac{\partial^2 W}{\partial t^2} \tag{2.6}$$

where ρ is the mass density of the cube and t is time. The left-hand side of the equation is the total force acting on the cube in the Z-direction, and the right-hand side is simply the product of the mass and the acceleration produced by the force.

2.2.1 Compressional wave

For the case where there are no shear stresses, κ_{zy} and $\kappa_{zx} = 0$, and Equation (2.6) can be reduced to

$$\frac{\partial \kappa_{zz}}{\partial z} = \rho\frac{\partial^2 W}{\partial t^2} \tag{2.7}$$

Substituting (2.3) into (2.7),

$$\frac{\partial^2 W}{\partial z^2} = \frac{\rho}{v + 2\mu}\frac{\partial^2 W}{\partial t^2} \tag{2.8}$$

This second-order differential equation is called the wave equation. The solutions for this equation have the form of $f(z \pm ct)$, where the negative sign indicates a wave traveling in the $+Z$-direction, whereas the positive sign indicates a wave traveling in the $-Z$-direction. The displacement W is in the same direction as the wave propagation, Z. This type of wave is called a compressional or longitudinal wave. The sinusoidal solution for this equation is

$$W^{\mp}(z,t) = W_0 e^{j(\omega t \pm kz)} \tag{2.9}$$

where W^- and W^+ denote displacements for positive and negative going waves, respectively, ω = angular frequency = $2\pi f$, $k = \omega/c$ is the wave number, and sound velocity c is given by

$$c = \sqrt{\frac{v + 2\mu}{\rho}} \tag{2.10}$$

For a fluid, μ can be assumed to approach 0; therefore,

$$c = \sqrt{\frac{B}{\rho}} = \sqrt{\frac{1}{G\rho}} \tag{2.11}$$

It is worth noting from this equation that the sound velocity in a medium is determined by the density and the compressibility of a medium. Sound velocity in air is much smaller than that in water. This is because although air has a small density, its compressibility is quite large, and thus offsets the smaller density.

2.2.2 *Shear wave*

For a case where $\kappa_{zz} = \kappa_{zy} = 0$, a new type of wave in which the displacement W is perpendicular to the direction of propagation X is characterized by

$$\frac{\partial \kappa_{zx}}{\partial x} = \rho \frac{\partial^2 W}{\partial t^2}$$

By substituting $\kappa_{zx} = \mu(\partial W/\partial x)$ into the equation above,

$$\frac{\partial^2 W}{\partial x^2} = \frac{\rho}{\mu} \frac{\partial^2 W}{\partial t^2} \tag{2.12}$$

This equation describes a wave traveling in the X-direction with a displacement in the Z-direction. The sinusoidal solution to Equation (2.12) is

$$W^{\mp}(x,t) = W_0 e^{j(\omega t \pm k_t x)} \qquad (2.13)$$

This type of wave expressed by (2.13) is called shear or transverse wave. The wave number for the shear wave is given by $k_t = \omega/c_t$, where c_t is the shear wave propagation velocity given by

$$c_t = \sqrt{\frac{\mu}{\rho}} \qquad (2.14)$$

It is obvious from Equation (2.14) that a shear wave can only exist in a medium with nonzero shear modulus; that is, fluid cannot support the propagation of a shear wave.

Both the longitudinal and shear velocities, as apparent from (2.11) and (2.14), are affected by the mechanical properties of a tissue. Pathological processes that alternate these properties can cause the sound velocity to change. Therefore, if the velocity of a tissue can be accurately measured, the result can be used to infer or diagnose its pathology. A few ultrasonic devices on the market today for diagnosing osteoporosis are based on this principle since osteoporosis causes a loss of bone mass.

2.3 *Characteristic impedance*

For sinusoidal excitation, the medium velocity or particle velocity in the Z-direction u_z can be found from the particle displacement W by differentiating W with respect to t:

$$u_z = \frac{\partial W}{\partial t} = j\omega W$$

It can be seen that the particle velocity is always 90° out of phase relative to the displacement. Since pressure is related to the stress by the following equation,

$$p = -\kappa_{zz}$$

it follows from (2.3) that

$$p = -(\nu + 2\mu)\frac{\partial W}{\partial z} \qquad (2.15)$$

For a longitudinal wave, the displacement W is given by (2.9). Substituting (2.9) into (2.15),

$$p^\pm = \pm jk(v + 2\mu)W^\pm = \pm j\omega\rho c W^\pm$$

Replacing $j\omega W$ by u_z,

$$p^\pm = \pm\rho c u_z{}^\pm \tag{2.16}$$

Note that the pressure, like the velocity, is 90° out of phase relative to the displacement. Equation (2.16) also indicates that the pressure and velocity are in phase for the positive-traveling wave, and 180° out of phase for the negative-traveling wave.

The specific acoustic impedance of a medium is defined as

$$Z^\pm = \frac{p^\pm}{u_z^\pm} = \pm\rho c \tag{2.17}$$

where the product ρc is also called the characteristic acoustic impedance of a medium. The acoustic impedance has a unit of kg/m²-s or Rayl to commemorate Lord Rayleigh, the father of modern acoustics. The positive and negative signs are for the positive and negative going waves, respectively. The acoustic velocity and impedance for a few common materials and biological tissues are listed in Table 2.1. The acoustic velocity in a medium is a sensitive function of the temperature, but its dependence on frequency is minimal over the frequency range from 1 to 15 MHz. As will

Table 2.1 Acoustic Properties of Biological Tissues and Relevant Materials

Material	Speed, m/s At 20–25°C	Acoustic impedance, MRayl	Attenuation coefficient, np/cm at 1 MHz	Backscattering coefficient, cm⁻¹sr⁻¹ at 5 MHz
Air	343	0.0004	1.38	—
Water	1480	1.48	0.00025	—
Fat	1450	1.38	0.06	—
Myocardium (perpendicular to fibers)	1550	1.62	0.35	8×10^{-4}
Blood	1550	1.61	0.02	2×10^{-5}
Liver	1570	1.65	0.11	5×10^{-3}
Skull bone	3360	6.00	1.30	—
Aluminum	6420	17.00	0.0021	—

be seen later, the acoustic impedance is a very important parameter in ultrasonic imaging since it determines the amplitude of the echoes that are reflected or scattered by tissue components. These echoes are acquired by an imaging device to form an image.

2.4 Intensity

The intensity of an ultrasonic wave is the average energy carried by a wave per unit area normal to the direction of propagation over time. It is well known that energy consumed by a force F that has moved an object by a distance L is equal to FL. The power is defined as energy per unit time. Since ultrasound is a pressure wave, intuitively one may deduce from the above relationship that the power, P, carried by an ultrasonic wave is given by

P = (Force exerted by the pressure wave · Medium displacement)/Time
= Force · Medium velocity

Now since intensity $i(t)$ is the power carried by the wave per unit area, it follows that

$$i(t) = dP/dA = p(t)u(t)$$

For the case of sinusoidal propagation, the average intensity I can be found by averaging $i(t)$ over a cycle:

$$I = p_0 u_0 \cdot \frac{1}{T} \int_0^T \sin^2 \omega t = \frac{1}{2} p_0 u_0 \tag{2.18}$$

where p_0 and u_0 denote peak values of pressure and medium velocity, and T is the period. Since $Z = p/u = \rho c$, substituting $p = \rho c u$ into (2.18),

$$I = \frac{1}{2} \rho c u_0^2$$

Here it is appropriate to define a few terms related to ultrasound intensity that have been used frequently in medical ultrasound as indicators of exposure level. These definitions are necessitated by the fact that a majority of the current ultrasonic imaging devices are of the pulse-echo type, in which very short pulses of ultrasound consisting of a few cycles of the oscillation are transmitted. This is illustrated in Figure 2.7. Therefore, the temporal averaged intensity differs from that given by Equation (2.18). Moreover, the intensity within an ultrasound beam in general is not spatially uniform. The typical profile of an ultrasonic beam is shown in Figure 2.8. The spatial

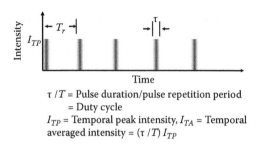

τ / T = Pulse duration/pulse repetition period
= Duty cycle
I_{TP} = Temporal peak intensity, I_{TA} = Temporal
averaged intensity = $(\tau / T) I_{TP}$

Figure 2.7 An ultrasonic pulse train in time with a temporal peak intensity I_{TP}, pulse duration τ, and pulse repetition period T.

averaged intensity I_{SA} is defined as the average intensity over the ultrasound beam.

$$I_{SA} = \frac{1}{A} \int_0^{\Delta r} I(r)\,dA$$

where $2\Delta r$ is the beam width, which is often defined as the spatial extent between the two -3 or -6 dB points, and A (the beam area) = $\pi\,(\Delta r)^2$. Figure 2.8 shows that the spatial peak intensity in the beam is 1 W/cm², while the spatial average intensity is only 0.8 W/cm².

Temporal average intensity is defined as the average intensity over a pulse repetition period T_r and is given by the product of duty factor and temporal peak intensity, where the duty factor is defined as

Duty factor = Pulsed duration (τ)/Pulsed repetition period (T_r)

Figure 2.7 shows that the duty factor is 0.2 in this case. Whenever biological effects of ultrasound are considered, it is absolutely crucial to state

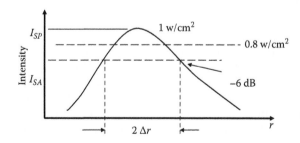

Figure 2.8 The ultrasonic lateral beam profile in the X-direction with the propagation direction in the Z-direction.

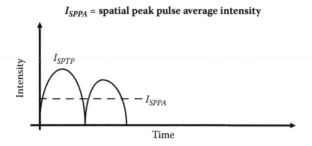

Figure 2.9 Definition of I_{SPPA}.

or understand which definition of intensity is being used (AIUM, 1984). In general, spatial average temporal average intensity I_{SATA} and spatial peak temporal average intensity I_{SPTA} are preferred. The U.S. Food and Drug Administration (FDA) also requires reporting a few other numbers when submitting an ultrasonic device for approval, including I_{SPPA}, spatial peak pulse-averaged intensity, and the total power emitted by a probe, depicted in Figure 2.9. The spatial peak pulse-averaged intensity is defined as the spatial peak intensity averaged over the pulse duration. As an example, a probe at 5 MHz emitting a total power of 1.1 mW at a pulse repetition frequency of 3 kHz may have an I_{SPTA} of 1.1 mW/cm², I_{SPPA} of 25 W/cm², and spatial peak and temporal peak pressure of 0.66 MPa at the focal point. These numbers indicate that the time-averaged intensity may be low, but the instantaneous peak pressure and intensity, which are concerns for mechanical bioeffects, can be very high. The potential bioeffects of ultrasound will be discussed in Chapter 10.

2.5 Acoustic radiation force

Like an optical wave, an acoustic wave exerts a body force called acoustic radiation force (ARF) to a medium due to the nonlinear interaction between ultrasound and the medium when there is a decrease in ultrasonic intensity in the direction of wave propagation (Nightingale, 2011). The ARF, f_r, is related to the intensity of the beam for a plane wave by the following equation:

$$f_r = \frac{2\alpha I}{c} \tag{2.19}$$

where I denotes intensity, c is sound velocity in the medium where the plane wave is propagating, and α is the attenuation coefficient of the medium. It has a unit of newton/m³. This can be found from Equation (2.19). The unit for $2\alpha I/c$ is $(1/m) \cdot (newton\text{-}m/s\text{-}m^2) \cdot (s/m) = newton/m^3$. The nonlinear interaction between ultrasound and a medium will be discussed in

Section 2.8 in more detail. Energy will be deposited into tissues as the wave penetrates deeper and harmonics are generated, resulting in a decrease in intensity and causing a force exerted on an object in the direction of wave propagation. This concept may be more easily understood from the particle point of view, i.e., a phonon in acoustics and a photon for optics. When a phonon or a photon collides with an object, e.g., a molecule, momentum transfer occurs and causes a force exerted on the object. The radiation force per unit area or radiation pressure p_r exerted by the wave on an object much larger than the wavelength is given by

$$p_r = a(I/c) \qquad\qquad (2.20)$$

where a is a constant depending upon the acoustic properties of the target and its geometry (Kossoff, 1972). If a target is made of a material of large acoustic impedance, such as steel, and reflects almost completely the ultrasound beam propagating in water, $a = 2$. If the target is a perfect absorber, $a = 1$. The reason for this can be understood by simply considering the momentum transfer that occurs as two objects collide, i.e.,

$$p_r \Delta t = \rho \Delta u$$

where ρ is the mass density, Δt is the contact time of the two objects, and Δu is the change in velocity of one of the two objects, assuming that the other is stationary. Since the momentum transfer that occurs at the interface for a perfect reflector is twice as large as that for an absorber, f_r acting on a perfect reflector should be twice as large. A more complete treatment can be found in Westervelt (1951).

The acoustic radiation force is a very useful phenomenon for determining power of an ultrasonic beam. A device that has often been used for measuring the intensity of an ultrasonic beam, called radiation force balance, is shown in Figure 2.10. A target with the surface covered with either an absorbing or a reflective material is suspended in water. The ultrasonic radiator should be positioned such that the beam is normally incident upon the target. The weight determined by the balance would yield the radiation pressure from which the intensity can be calculated using Equation (2.20).

The acoustic radiation force has been used as a means to perturb an object remotely so that from the displacement of the object, which can be measured via ultrasonic imaging, an assessment of the elastic properties of the medium surrounding the object may be made (Nightingale, 2011).

2.6 Reflection and refraction

As a plane ultrasonic wave encounters an interface between two media, I and II, of different acoustic impedance, it will be reflected and refracted. Part of the energy carried by the incident wave is reflected and travels at the

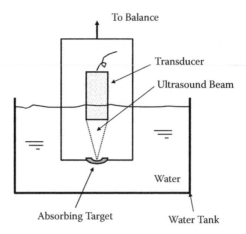

Figure 2.10 A radiation balance with an absorbing target.

same velocity as the incident wave. The transmitted or refracted wave in the second medium travels at a different velocity. The directions of the reflected and refracted waves are governed, just as in optics, by Snell's law. This is illustrated in Figure 2.11, where the subscripts *i*, *r*, and *t* refer to incident, reflected, and transmitted or refracted waves, respectively. The boundary conditions are that the pressure and medium velocity must be continuous, and the energy is conserved across the boundary, that is, at the boundary:

$$p_i + p_r = p_t$$

$$u_i + u_r = u_t$$

$$I_i = I_r + I_t$$

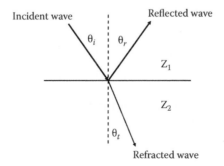

Figure 2.11 A plane ultrasonic wave reflected and refracted by a flat interface between two media.

By applying these relationships, it is found that as in optics,

$$\theta_i = \theta_r \quad \text{and} \quad \sin\theta_i/\sin\theta_t = c_1/c_2 \tag{2.21}$$

where $\theta_t = \pi/2$, $\sin\theta_t = 1$, and $\theta_{ic} = \sin^{-1}(c_1/c_2)$ if $c_2 > c_1$. For any incident angle greater than θ_{ic}, there is no transmission; that is, total reflection occurs. Therefore, θ_{ic} is called the critical angle.

The pressure reflection and transmission coefficients, R and T, can be easily found by using the boundary conditions that the pressure and particle velocity should be continuous across the boundary.

$$R = \frac{p_r}{p_i} = \frac{Z_2 \cos\theta_i - Z_1 \cos\theta_t}{Z_2 \cos\theta_i + Z_1 \cos\theta_t} \tag{2.22}$$

$$T = \frac{p_t}{p_i} = \frac{2Z_2 \cos\theta_i}{Z_2 \cos\theta_i + Z_1 \cos\theta_t} \tag{2.23}$$

For normal incidence, $\theta_i = \theta_t = 0$, and (2.22) and (2.23) become

$$R = p_r/p_i = (Z_2 - Z_1)/(Z_2 + Z_1) \tag{2.24}$$

$$T = p_t/p_i = 2Z_2/(Z_2 + Z_1) \tag{2.25}$$

Since $p = Zu$, $I = p_o^2/2Z$, from Equations (2.22) and (2.23), it can be shown that,

$$\frac{I_r}{I_i} = \left(\frac{Z_2 \cos\theta_i - Z_1 \cos\theta_t}{Z_2 \cos\theta_i + Z_1 \cos\theta_t}\right)^2 \tag{2.26}$$

$$\frac{I_t}{I_i} = \frac{4Z_2 Z_1 \cos\theta_i}{(Z_2 \cos\theta_i + Z_1 \cos\theta_t)^2} \tag{2.27}$$

The quantities (I_r/I_i) and (I_t/I_i) are, respectively, intensity reflection and transmission coefficients at the interface. For normal incidence, $\theta_i = \theta_t = 0$, (2.26) and (2.27) become

$$I_r/I_i = [(Z_2 - Z_1)/(Z_2 + Z_1)]^2 \tag{2.28}$$

$$I_t/I_i = 4Z_2 Z_1/(Z_2 + Z_1)^2 \tag{2.29}$$

As an acoustic wave propagates through an inhomogeneous medium such as biological tissues, part of its energy will be lost due to absorption and scattering, which will be discussed later, and part of its energy will be lost due to specular reflection at the boundary of two adjacent layers of tissues. The ultrasonic images are formed from the specularly reflected echoes due to planar interfaces as well as the diffusely scattered echoes due to small inhomogeneities in tissue parenchyma. Therefore, any change in the elastic properties of the tissues as a result of a disease may be detectable from the ultrasonic image. This has been the principal rationale behind the conventional pulse-echo ultrasonic imaging methods. Since both scattering and reflection depend on the elastic properties of the tissues, which determine the acoustic impedance of the tissue, intuitively one may postulate that echographic visualizability of tissues is determined mostly by their connective tissue content (Fields and Dunn, 1973). The acoustic impedance of connective tissues and tissues containing high concentrations of connective tissues has been found to be much higher than other types of tissue components, such as fat and protein and tissues containing less connective tissues. The velocity in collagen has been found to be approximately $1.7 \cdot 10^5$ cm/s (Goss and O'Brien, 1979). The acoustic impedance of blood vessels, which are composed mainly of connective tissues, should be and was found to be higher than that of most other tissues (Geleski and Shung, 1982). Because of their higher impedance than surrounding tissues, tissues that contain more connective tissues should be more echogenic than those that contain less. However, it must be noted that the attenuation of ultrasound in connective tissues is also much higher (Greenleaf, 1986). Very little energy can transmit through a mass such as a solid tumor composed of mainly connective tissues. Thus, an acoustic shadow may be created behind such a mass. This has been used as one of the criteria for diagnosing tumors. The origin of the ultrasonic echoes observed in an ultrasonic image for most of the soft tissues has not yet been determined. There is, however, experimental evidence suggesting that at least in muscle and myocardium, the collagen fibers surrounding the muscle fibers affect to a great extent the echogenicity of these tissues (Hete and Shung, 1993). Although the postulation that tissue echogenicity is largely determined by its connective tissue content may appear to be true, other factors, such as cellular dimension and tissue complexity, should also play an important role and cannot be ignored (Shung and Thieme, 1993). There has been a long-standing interest in correlating the acoustic parameters, such as scattering, attenuation, and acoustic impedance, to the biological composition of the tissues or ultrasonic characterization of biological tissues (Greenleaf, 1986; Shung and Thieme, 1993).

2.7 Attenuation, absorption, and scattering

When an ultrasonic wave propagates through a heterogeneous medium, its energy is reduced or attenuated as a function of distance. The energy may be diverted by reflection or scattering or absorbed by the medium and converted to heat. The reflection and scattering of a wave by an object actually are referring to the same phenomenon, the redistribution of the energy from the primary incident direction into other directions. This redistribution of energy is termed reflection when the wavelength and wavefront of the wave are much smaller than the object, and is termed scattering if the wavelength and the wavefront are greater than or comparable to the dimension of the object.

2.7.1 Attenuation

The pressure of a plane monochromatic wave propagating in the Z-direction decreases exponentially as a function of z:

$$p(z) = p(z = 0)e^{-\alpha z} \qquad (2.30)$$

where $p(z = 0)$ is the pressure at $z = 0$ and α is the pressure attenuation coefficient.

Therefore,

$$\alpha = \frac{1}{z} \ln \left[\frac{p(z = 0)}{p(z)} \right]$$

The attenuation coefficient has a unit of np/cm and is sometimes expressed in the unit of dB/cm, or

$$\alpha(\text{dB/cm}) = 20(\log_{10} e)\alpha(\text{np/cm}) = 8.686\alpha(\text{np/cm})$$

To convert α in np/cm to dB/cm, simply multiply α in np/cm by 8.686. If a tissue has an attenuation coefficient of 0.1 np/cm, in dB/cm, $\alpha = 8.686 \times 0.1$ dB/cm = 0.8686 dB/cm. Typical values of the attenuation coefficient in some materials are given in Table 2.1.

The relative importance of absorption and scattering to attenuation of ultrasound in biological tissues is a matter being continuously debated. Investigations to date have shown that scattering contributes little to attenuation, at most a few percent, in most soft tissues (Shung and Thieme, 1993). Therefore, it is safe to say that absorption is the dominant mechanism for ultrasonic attenuation in biological tissues.

2.7.2 Absorption

As was discussed earlier, part of the ultrasound energy propagating in an inhomogeneous medium is lost due to the redistribution of the energy, such as scattering and reflection, and part of the energy is absorbed by the medium. The energy absorbed by the medium is converted to heat. The absorption mechanisms in biological tissues are quite complex and have been assumed to arise from (1) classical absorption due to viscosity and (2) a relaxation phenomenon. Both mechanisms depend upon the frequency of the wave. In earlier developments an ideal fluid with $\mu \sim 0$ has been assumed, and this means that the absorption due to the classical viscous loss is ignored. However, in reality, this is seldom the case. Recall the definition of shear strain in the X-direction along the Z-axis:

$$\varepsilon_{xz} = \frac{\partial U}{\partial z}$$

In fluids, the rate of strain, which is of more interest than the strain itself, is given by

$$\frac{\partial \varepsilon_{xz}}{\partial t} = \frac{\partial}{\partial t}\frac{\partial U}{\partial z} = \frac{\partial u_x}{\partial z} \tag{2.31}$$

where u_x is the particle velocity in the X-direction and $\partial u_x/\partial z$ is the velocity gradient along the Z-axis. When a fluid with finite viscosity is subject to shear stress, κ_{xz}, as shown in Figure 2.12, it exhibits a velocity gradient, $\partial u_x/\partial z$. The coefficient of viscosity, denoted as η with a unit in poises, is defined as the ratio of shear stress to the resultant velocity gradient:

$$\eta = \frac{\kappa_{xz}}{\partial u_x / \partial z} \tag{2.32}$$

It has been shown that for a homogeneous medium like water, the absorption coefficient for an ultrasonic wave of frequency ω is related to viscosity and frequency by the following expression:

$$\alpha = \frac{2\omega^2 \eta}{3\rho c}$$

where $\eta = \mu/j\omega$ from Equations (2.5) and (2.32). Note here that the absorption coefficient is proportional to ω^2. In many homogeneous materials, such as air and water, where the elemental particles of the medium are

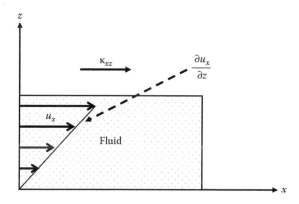

Figure 2.12 Shear stress in the X-direction on a Z-plane produces a velocity gradient along the Z-direction.

much smaller than the wavelength, this (frequency)^2 dependence of absorption is seen, but in most biological materials, this is not the case. Experimental results on the attenuation coefficient of ultrasound in biological tissues indicate an approximately linear dependence on frequency below 15 MHz, and an alternative theory is needed to explain this behavior. It has been theorized that ultrasonic absorption in biological tissues is dominated by a relaxation process.

When an elemental particle in a medium such as a molecule is pushed to a new position by a force and then released, a finite time is required for the particle to return to its neutral position. This time is called the relaxation time of the particle. For a medium that is composed of the same type of particles, the relaxation time is also the relaxation time of the medium. If the relaxation time is short compared to the period of the wave, its effect on the wave should be small. However, if the relaxation time is comparable to the period of the wave, the particle may not be able to completely return to its neutral state before a second wave arrives. When this occurs, the wave is moving in one direction, whereas the molecules are moving in the other direction. More energy is thus required to reverse the direction of the particle motion. If the frequency is increased high enough that the molecules simply cannot follow the wave motion, the relaxation effect again becomes negligible. Maximum absorption occurs when the relaxation motion of the particles is completely out of synchronization with the wave motion. Therefore, the relaxation process is characterized by a relaxation frequency where the absorption is maximal and is negligibly small for low-frequency and high-frequency regions, illustrated in Figure 2.13. Mathematically, the relaxation process can be represented by the following equation:

$$\alpha_r = \frac{Bf^2}{1+(f/f_R)^2}$$

where α_r = component of the absorption coefficient due to the relaxation process, f_R = relaxation frequency = $1/T_R$, T_R = relaxation time, and B is a

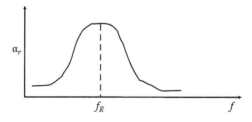

Figure 2.13 Ultrasonic absorption caused by a relaxation process characterized by relaxation frequency f_R.

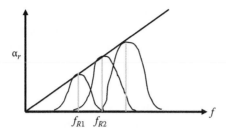

Figure 2.14 Ultrasonic absorption caused by multiple relaxation processes characterized by relaxation frequency $f_{R1}, f_{R2}, \ldots$

constant. In a biological tissue, there are many components, giving rise to many relaxation frequencies. The absorption coefficient in a tissue can be expressed as

$$\alpha_a / f^2 = A + \sum_i \frac{B_i}{1 + (f/f_{Ri})^2} \tag{2.33}$$

where A is a constant associated with classical absorption and B_i and f_{Ri} are the relaxation constants and frequencies associated with different tissue components (Dunn and Goss, 1986). A possible scenario for this equation is illustrated in Figure 2.14, where many relaxation processes may overlap, resulting in a linear increase in the diagnostic ultrasound frequency range or a constant $\alpha\lambda$. Figure 2.15 shows the absorption of ultrasound in various biological tissues as a function of frequency. As can be seen, the absorption

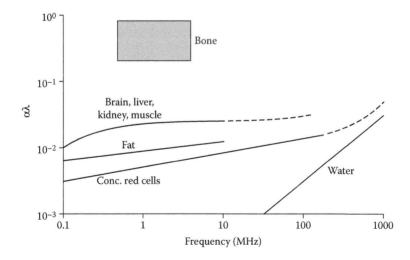

Figure 2.15 Ultrasonic absorption in biological tissues as a function of frequency.

is more or less linearly proportional to frequency ($\alpha\lambda$ is constant) in the diagnostic ultrasound frequency range. Also in this figure, it can be seen that the absorption of ultrasound in water is proportional to f^2.

2.7.3 Scattering

As a wave is incident on an object, as shown in Figure 2.16, part of the wave will be scattered and part of the wave will be absorbed by the object. The scattering characteristics are most conveniently expressed by a term called scattering cross section.

Assume that the incident pressure is a plane monochromatic wave $p_i(r) = e^{-j\mathbf{k}\cdot\mathbf{r}}$, where $\mathbf{k} = k\mathbf{i}$ (**i** denotes a unit vector in the incident direction) and **r** are vectors representing the wave number and the position, respectively. The scattered wave at $\mathbf{r_s}$ due to a scatterer at $\mathbf{r_0}$ is given by

$$p_s(\mathbf{r_s}) = \frac{e^{-jkR}}{R} p_i(\mathbf{r_0}) f(\mathbf{o},\mathbf{i}) \tag{2.34}$$

where **o** is a unit vector in the direction of observation, provided that the observation point is in the far field of the scatterer and $R = |\mathbf{r_s} - \mathbf{r_0}|$ if $kR \gg 1$. The term $f(\mathbf{o},\mathbf{i})$ in (2.34) is called the scattering amplitude function, which describes the scattering properties of the object and depends upon the directions of incidence and observation. The incident intensity in a medium of acoustic impedance Z is given by

$$I_i = \frac{1}{2}\frac{|p_i|^2}{Z} \tag{2.35}$$

and the scattered intensity is given by

$$I_s = \frac{1}{2}\frac{|p_s|^2}{Z} \tag{2.36}$$

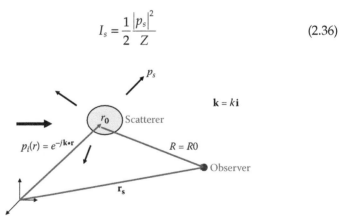

Figure 2.16 A plane wave incident upon a scatterer.

Substituting (2.34) and (2.35) into (2.36) and rearranging the equation,

$$I_s = \frac{|f(\mathbf{o},\mathbf{i})|^2}{R^2} I_i \tag{2.37}$$

Rearranging (2.36),

$$\sigma_d(\mathbf{o},\mathbf{i}) = |f(\mathbf{o},\mathbf{i})|^2 = \frac{I_s R^2}{I_i} \tag{2.38}$$

where the term $\sigma_d(\mathbf{o},\mathbf{i}) = |f|^2$ is defined as the differential scattering cross section, which is the power scattered in the **o**-direction with the incident direction **i** in one solid angle per unit incident intensity. When $\mathbf{o} = -\mathbf{i}$, $\sigma_d(\mathbf{i},-\mathbf{i})$ is called the backscattering cross section. Figure 2.17 gives a graphical illustration of differential scattering cross section. By integrating σ_d over the 4π solid angle, the scattering cross section σ_s, which is defined as the power scattered by the object per unit incident intensity, can be found.

$$\sigma_s = \int_{4\pi} \sigma_d \, d\Omega = \int_{4\pi} |f(\mathbf{o},\mathbf{i})|^2 \, d\Omega$$

where $d\Omega$ is the differential solid angle. Similarly, an absorption cross section, σ_a, can be defined as the total power absorbed by the object.

Differential scattering cross section $\sigma_d(\mathbf{i},\mathbf{o})$: power scattered in one solid angle in **o** direction per unit incident intensity in **i** direction

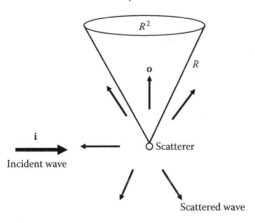

Figure 2.17 The differential scattering cross section of a scatterer represents the power scattered by the scatterer into one solid angle or steradian that encompasses an area of R^2.

Thus, the attenuation in wave intensity due to the presence of the object is simply

$$2\alpha = \sigma_a + \sigma_s$$

where 2α is the intensity attenuation coefficient. If there are a number of objects, the intensity attenuation coefficient should be

$$2\alpha = n(\sigma_a + \sigma_s)$$

where n is the object concentration per unit volume. This relation is valid only if n is small or volume concentration given by $n \cdot$ (object volume) < 1%. As n increases, multiple scattering occurs and there may be particle–particle interactions (Twersky, 1978), and this relation no longer holds.

To solve analytically for the scattering cross section of an object of arbitrary shape is impossible, although there are computer-based methods such as finite element analysis that may be used. However, a number of approximations exist that can simplify the problem considerably. One of these is the Born approximation, which assumes that the wave inside the object is the same as the incident wave (Morse and Ingard, 1968). This is a valid assumption if the size of the object is much smaller than the wavelength, or the acoustic properties of the scatterer are similar to those of the surrounding medium. By applying this approximation and using the wave equation, the scattering cross section of an object can be found. The scattering cross section for a sphere whose radius is much smaller than the wavelength is given by (Morse and Ingard, 1968)

$$\sigma_s = \frac{4\pi k^4 a^6}{9}\left(\left|\frac{G_e - G}{G}\right|^2 + \frac{1}{3}\left|\frac{3\rho_e - 3\rho}{2\rho_e + \rho}\right|^2\right) \tag{2.39}$$

where k is the wave number, a is the radius of the sphere, G_e and G are the adiabatic compressibilities of the particle and the surrounding medium, and ρ_e and ρ are the corresponding mass densities. Equation (2.39) can be applied to calculating the ultrasonic scattering properties of the red blood cells since the size of a red cell is much smaller than the wavelength of ultrasound in the frequency range from 1 to 15 MHz. Assume that the human red blood can be approximated as a fluid sphere of 3 μm radius. Using G_e (compressibility for red blood cell) = $34.1 \cdot 10^{-12}$ cm²/dyne, ρ_e (density for the red blood cell) = 1.092 gm/cm³, G (compressibility for plasma) = $40.9 \cdot 10^{-12}$ cm²/dyne, and ρ (density for plasma) = 1.021 gm/cm³, the scattering cross section for a red cell is found to be $\sigma_s = 1.1 \cdot 10^{-12}$ cm² at 10 MHz, which is quite small. For an incident intensity of 1 W/cm², only $\sigma_s \cdot I_i = 1.1 \cdot 10^{-12}$ W is scattered by the red cell.

In a dense distribution of scatterers like biological tissues, for instance, human blood consisting of $5 \cdot 10^9$ red blood cells in 1 cm³, scatterer-to-scatterer interaction cannot be ignored. To take this into consideration, a parameter called backscattering coefficient in a unit of (cm-steradian)$^{-1}$ is often used. It is also sometimes called volumetric backscattering cross section and is defined as the power backscattered by a unit volume of scatterers in one solid angle per unit incident intensity. The physical meaning of the backscattering coefficient can be easily understood simply by replacing the scatterer in Figure 2.17 by a unit scattering volume. Since the tissues are fairly inhomogeneous, the scattered signals acquired may vary greatly at any single frequency and over a band of frequencies; a parameter that is frequently used to describe scattering behavior of a tissue is the integrated backscatter. The integrated backscatter (IB) is defined as the frequency average of the backscatter over the bandwidth of the signal, which mathematically can be expressed as

$$IB = \frac{1}{2\Delta\omega} \int_{\omega_0 - \Delta\omega}^{\omega_0 + \Delta\omega} e(\omega) d\omega$$

where $2\Delta\omega$ is the bandwidth, ω_0 is the center frequency of the spectrum, and $e(\omega)$ is the backscattered signal at angular frequency ω. However, in order to eliminate the dependence of the backscattered signal from tissues on the electrical and acoustic characteristics of the experimental system, the *IB* is usually expressed in dB by comparing the backscattered signal to a reference signal, e.g., the echo from a flat reflector.

Therefore,

$$IB(dB) = 20\log\left[\int_{\omega_0 - \Delta\omega}^{\omega_0 + \Delta\omega} e(\omega) d\omega \bigg/ \int_{\omega_0 - \Delta\omega}^{\omega_0 + \Delta\omega} e_r(\omega) d\omega \right]$$

where $e_r(\omega)$ is the reflected signal from the flat reflector at angular frequency ω. The backscattering coefficient for several tissues is listed in Table 2.1.

The fact that the acoustic scattering characteristics of an object, including angular scattering pattern, depend upon the shape, size, and acoustic properties of the scatterer has been known for many years. Ideally, the structure and acoustic properties of the scatterers can be deduced from measuring their scattering properties. This problem is of interest to many scientists in such diverse fields as geophysics, oceanography, and communication. It is generally termed remote sensing or detection. Although the potential of characterizing a tissue structure from its scattering properties was realized in the biomedical ultrasound community almost three decades ago, this field still remains in its infancy, primarily due to the complex nature of biological tissues. Preliminary experimental investigations *in vitro* so far have shown that different tissues exhibit different angular scattering patterns and frequency dependence (Shung and Thieme, 1993). The backscattering coefficient defined as backscattering cross section per unit volume of scatterers for five different types of bovine tissues as a function of frequency is shown in Figure 2.18 (Fei and Shung, 1985). Experimental results on scattering by red blood cells (Yuan and Shung, 1988) are in good agreement with Equation (2.39). Scattering from the myocardium has been shown to have a third power dependence on frequency (Shung and Thieme, 1993). Based on this evidence and more recent results indicating that ultrasonic scattering increases as the muscle is stretched, it was suggested that the scattering from muscle

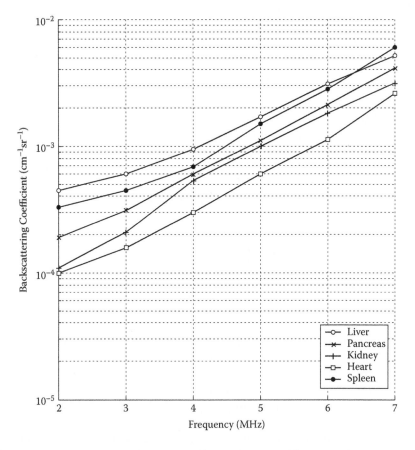

Figure 2.18 Ultrasonic backscatter coefficient for several bovine soft tissues as a function of frequency.

may be attributed to the collagen fibers in the muscle, because the scattering from cylinders whose radius is much smaller than the wavelength is proportional to f^3. Experimental results on scattering from tissues thus far have been very scanty and inconclusive. The precise origin of ultrasonic scattering from many tissues is still unknown, although there are efforts underway to shed more light on this subject (Shung and Thieme, 1993).

Since pathological processes in tissues involve anatomical variations, it is likely that they will result in corresponding changes in ultrasonic backscatter. This has been demonstrated by several recent investigations. Figure 2.19 shows that the backscattering coefficient for regions of infarcted myocardium is substantially higher than that for normal myocardium (Wickline et al., 1993). In addition, rnyocardial ultrasonic backscatter is shown to be related to the contractional state of the tissue (Figure 2.20). The myocardial backscatter was found to

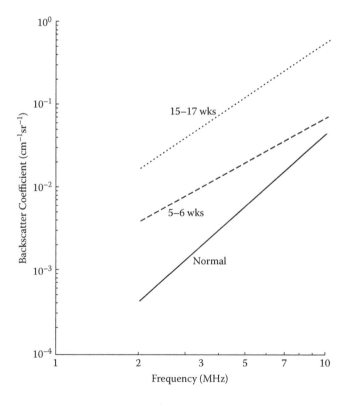

Figure 2.19 Ultrasonic backscatter coefficient for canine myocardium as a function of frequency. Solid, dashed, and dotted lines represent data for normal myocardium, myocardium 5–6 weeks following infarction, and myocardium 15 to 17 weeks following infarction, respectively.

be the highest at end diastole and the lowest at end systole during a cardiac cycle, and this cyclic behavior was blunted in ischemic heart (Wickline et al., 1993).

In summary, the attenuation of ultrasound in biological tissues can be attributed to two mechanisms: (1) scattering and (2) absorption. The question remains, however, as to the relative importance of these mechanisms, although absorption is believed to be the dominant mechanism. Attenuation in general is not desirable because it limits the depth of penetration ultrasound into the body. However, it may yield useful information for diagnostic purposes because it carries information about the properties of the tissues if it can be accurately estimated. Extensive work has also been carried out to demonstrate that tissue pathology can affect

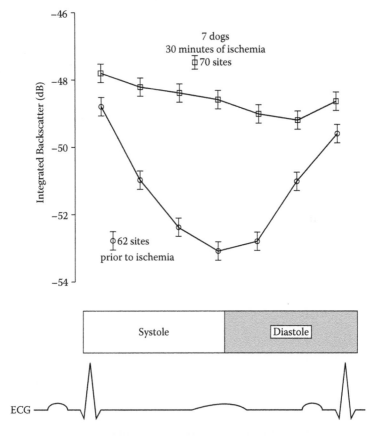

Figure 2.20 Integrated backscatter from canine myocardium as a function of the cardiac cycle.

to a great extent the attenuation coefficient of tissues. Infarcted myocardium and malignant tumors in liver and breast were all shown to have an increased attenuation. Unfortunately, measuring attenuation *in vivo* has proven to be a quite difficult task. Various schemes have been developed with little success.

2.8 Nonlinearity parameter B/A

Since the spatial peak temporal peak intensity I_{SPTP} of modern ultrasonic diagnostic instruments can sometimes reach the level of more than 100 W/cm^2 and the peak pressure level can reach a few Mpascals (one atmospheric pressure is 0.1 Mpascal), nonlinear acoustic phenomena may not be ignored in treating ultrasonic propagation in tissues (Hamilton and Blackstock, 1998). Although finite amplitude acoustics has been in existence for a long time, it has not been given much attention in diagnostic ultrasound until recently, when harmonic imaging became popular (Tranquart et al., 1999). In fact, it has been shown that in many instances harmonic imaging that utilizes the harmonics generated due to the nonlinear propagation yields better images than conventional ultrasonic imaging. Other reasons for studying the nonlinear properties are: (1) new tissue parameters may be derived for tissue characterization and (2) nonlinearity can influence, to a significant extent, how the ultrasound energy is absorbed by the tissue.

The nonlinear behavior of a fluid medium can be expressed by a second-order parameter B/A. For an adiabatic process in which the entropy is constant or there is no energy flow, the relation between pressure and density can be expressed as a Taylor series expansion of pressure, p, about the point of equilibrium density, ρ_0, and entropy, s_0,

$$p = p(s_0, \rho_0) + A\left(\frac{\rho - \rho_0}{\rho_0}\right) + \frac{1}{2}B\left(\frac{\rho - \rho_0}{\rho_0}\right)^2 + \cdots$$

where

$$A = \rho_0 \left[\frac{\partial p(s_0, \rho_0)}{\partial \rho}\right]$$

and

$$B = \rho_0^2 \left[\frac{\partial^2 p(s_0, \rho_0)}{\partial \rho^2}\right]$$

From these two equations and the definition of sound speed (Morse and Ingard, 1968),

$$c^2 = \frac{\partial p(s_0, \rho_0)}{\partial \rho}$$

we can show that B/A is given by

$$B/A = 2\rho_0 c_0 \left[\frac{\partial c(s_0, \rho_0)}{\partial p} \right] \tag{2.40}$$

Equation (2.40) can be converted to parameters that are easier to measure using thermodynamic relationships:

$$B/A = 2\rho_0 c_0 \left[\frac{\partial c(s, T)}{\partial p} \right] + 2 \frac{c_0 T \beta_v}{C_p} \left[\frac{\partial c(s, p)}{\partial T} \right] \tag{2.41}$$

where T is temperature, C_p is the heat capacity per unit mass at constant pressure, and β_v is the volume coefficient of thermal expansion. The first term represents change in sound speed per unit change in pressure at constant temperature and entropy. The second term represents the change in sound speed per unit change in temperature at constant pressure and entropy. Therefore, the B/A parameter can be estimated from these quantities, which are either known or measurable. This approach is called the thermodynamic method. It can also be estimated by a finite amplitude method in which the second pressure harmonic is measured and extrapolated back to the source to eliminate the effect of absorption. The preliminary findings are (1) B/A is linearly proportional to the solute concentration in aqueous solutions of proteins, (2) B/A is insensitive to the molecular weight of the solute at fixed concentrations, (3) B/A ranges from 6 to 11 for soft tissues, and (4) B/A may be dependent upon tissue structure. The B/A values for a few tissues and relevant materials are given in Table 2.2.

Table 2.2 B/A Values for Various Materials

Material	B/A
Water	5.0 at 20°C
Bovine serum albumin (20 g/100 ml)	6.2 at 25°C
Beef liver	7.8 at 23°C
Human breast fat	9.2 at 22°C
Porcine muscle	6.5 at 25°C
Porcine whole blood	6.2 at 30°C

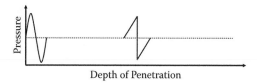

Depth of Penetration

Figure 2.21 Wave distortion resulting from the nonlinear interaction between ultrasound and the medium.

The nonlinearity of ultrasonic wave propagation can cause the distortion of waveforms as illustrated in Figure 2.21, which shows that a sinusoidal waveform becomes a sawtooth waveform, as a result of the generation of higher harmonics after propagating in a medium. This is plausible in that the velocity in a denser region of the medium should be greater. The harmonic amplitudes relative to that at the fundamental or first harmonic frequency as a function of the normalized propagation distance z/z_1 are shown in Figure 2.22, where $z_1 = \rho c^2 / [(1 + 0.5B/A)kp_0]$ (Pierce, 1986). Here k is the wave number and p_0 is the peak pressure. It is clear that the amplitude of the fundamental frequency drops and the

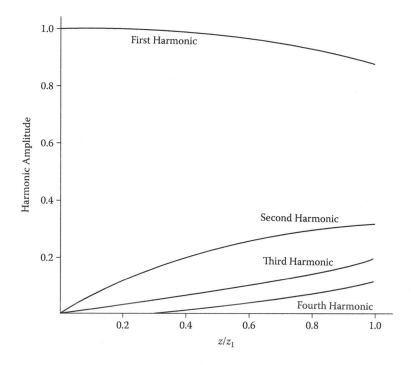

Figure 2.22 Harmonic amplitude as a function of the normalized depth of penetration as a plane acoustic wave propagates into a liquid medium.

amplitudes of higher harmonics increase as the propagation distance increases.

2.9 Doppler effect

The Doppler effect describes a phenomenon in which a change in the frequency of sound emitted from a source is perceived by an observer when the source or the observer is moving or both are moving. The reason for the perceived frequency change for a moving source and a stationary observer is illustrated in Figure 2.23. In diagram (a), the sound source Sp is stationary and producing a uniform spherical spreading of the wave, and the frequency of the sound perceived by an observer is $f = c/\lambda$, where c is the velocity of sound in the medium and λ is the wavelength, shown as the distance between two crests. In diagram (b), the sound source is moving to the right at a velocity v. The source motion changes the distance between the crests, increasing frequency and decreasing the wavelength to the right, and decreasing the frequency and increasing the wavelength to the left. The frequency perceived by an observer on the right is

$$f' = \frac{c}{\lambda'} = \frac{c}{\lambda - vT} = \frac{c}{(c-v)T} = \frac{c}{c-v}f$$

and the frequency seen by an observer on the left is

$$f' = \frac{c}{c+v}f$$

The difference between the actual frequency of the source f and the perceived frequency f' is called the Doppler frequency, f_d. A similar relationship can also be obtained for a moving observer. When combining these relationships, for a source moving with a velocity v and an observer with velocity v', the Doppler frequency can be found to be given by

$$f_d = f' - f = \left(\frac{c+v'}{c-v} - 1\right)f \qquad (2.42)$$

If both the source and observer are moving at the same velocity, v, assuming $c \gg v$, then Equation (2.42) can be reduced to

$$f_d = \frac{2vf}{c} \qquad (2.43)$$

Doppler effect

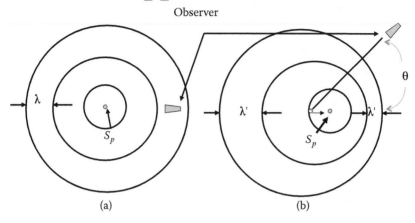

Observer

(a)   (b)

Figure 2.23 A stationary observer perceives a change in frequency of a wave emitted by a moving source toward the observer resulting from a change in wavelength from λ to λ'. (a) The source is stationary. (b) The source is moving at a velocity v.

For the situation where the velocity is making an angle of θ relative to the direction of sound propagation, as shown in Figure 2.23(b), v in Equation (2.43) should be replaced by $v(\cos\theta)$:

$$f_d = \frac{2v(\cos\theta)f}{c} \tag{2.44}$$

The Doppler effect is used in ultrasonic Doppler devices for the measurement and imaging of blood flow transcutaneously, i.e., without penetrating the skin in any manner. In these devices ultrasonic waves are launched into a blood vessel by an ultrasonic transducer, and the scattered radiation from the moving red cells is detected by either the same transducer or a separate transducer. Appropriate instrumentation is incorporated to extract the Doppler frequency, which is proportional to the red cell velocity.

References and Further Reading Materials

American Institute of Ultrasound in Medicine. *Safety considerations for diagnostic ultrasound*. Laurel, MD: AIUM, 1984.

Dunn F and Goss SA. Definitions of terms and measurements of acoustical quantities. In Greenleaf JF (ed.), *Tissue characterization with ultrasound*. Boca Raton, FL: CRC Press, 1986, pp. 1–14.

Fei DY and Shung KK. Ultrasonic backscatter from mammalian tissues. *J Acoust Soc Am* 1985; 78: 871–877.

Fields S and Dunn F. Correlation of echographic visualizability of tissue with biological composition and physiological state. *J Acoust Soc Am* 1973; 54: 809–811.

Geleskie JV and Shung KK. Further studies on the acoustic impedance of major bovine blood vessel walls. *J Acoust Soc Am* 1982; 71: 467–470.

Goss SA and O'Brien WD Jr. Direct ultrasonic velocity measurements of mammalian collagen threads. *J Acoust Soc Am* 1979; 65: 507–511.

Greenleaf JA. *Tissue characterization with ultrasound.* Boca Raton, FL: CRC Press, 1986.

Hamilton MF and Blackstock DT. *Nonlinear acoustics.* San Diego: Academic Press, 1998.

Hete B and Shung KK. Scattering of ultrasound from skeletal muscle tissue. *IEEE Trans Ultrasonics Ferroelect Freq Cont* 1993; 40: 354–365.

Kossoff G. Radiation force. In Reid JM and Sikov MR (eds.), *Interaction of ultrasound and biological tissues.* Rockville, MD: FDA, 1972, pp. 159–161.

Malecki I. *Physical foundations of technical acoustics.* New York: Pergman Press, 1969.

Morse PM and Ingard KU. *Theoretical acoustics.* New York: McGraw Hill, 1968.

Nightingale K. Acoustic radiation force impulse (ARFI) imaging: A review. *Curr Med Imaging Rev* 2011; 7: 328–339.

Pierce A. *Acoustics: An introduction to physical principles and applications.* New York: McGraw Hill, 1986.

Shung KK and Thieme GA. *Ultrasonic scattering by biological tissues.* Boca Raton, FL: CRC Press, 1993.

Tranquart F, Grenier N, Eder V, and Pourcelot L. Clinical use of ultrasound tissue harmonic imaging. *Ultrasonics Med Biol* 1999; 25: 889–894.

Twersky V. Acoustic bulk parameters in distributions of pair-correlated scatterers. *J Acoust Soc Am* 1978; 64: 1710–1719.

Westervelt PJ. The theory of steady forces caused by sound waves. *J Acoust Soc Am* 1951; 23: 312–315.

Wickline SA, Perez JE, and Miller JG. Cardiovascular tissue characterization in vivo. In Shung KK and Thieme GA (eds.), *Ultrasonic scattering in biological tissues.* Boca Raton, FL: CRC Press, 1993, pp. 313–345.

Yuan YW and Shung KK. Ultrasonic backscatter from flowing whole blood. I. Dependence on shear rate and hematocrit. *J Acoust Soc Am* 1988; 84: 52–58.

chapter three

Ultrasonic transducers and arrays

All ultrasonic imaging systems require a device called an ultrasonic transducer to convert electrical energy into ultrasonic or acoustic energy and vice versa. Ultrasonic transducers come in a variety of forms and sizes, ranging from single-element transducers for mechanical scanning to linear arrays to multidimensional arrays for electronic scanning. Although the performance of an ultrasonic scanner is critically dependent upon transducers/arrays, array/transducer performance has been one of the bottlenecks that has prevented current ultrasonic imagers from reaching their theoretical resolution limit. The primary reason is that medical ultrasonic array/transducer design and fabrication are processes of a broad interdisciplinary nature. They require knowledge from a variety of disciplines, such as acoustics and vibration, electrical engineering, material sciences and engineering, medical imaging, and anatomy and physiology. It is no wonder that even to date the design of transducers is still mostly empirical, generally involving a trial-and-error approach. Many manufacturers regard their expertise in designing and manufacturing transducers as a trade secret of the highest order.

The most critical component of an ultrasonic transducer is a piezoelectric element.

3.1 Piezoelectric effect

The phenomenon that a material upon the application of an electrical field changes its physical dimensions and vice versa is known as the piezoelectric effect (pressure-electric effect) (Cady, 1964; Kino, 1987). The piezoelectric effect was discovered by French physicists Pierre and Jacques Curie in 1880. The direct and reverse piezoelectric effects are illustrated in Figure 3.1(a) and (b), respectively. The direct effect refers to the phenomenon in which the application of a stress causes a net charge to appear across the electrodes, whereas the inverse effect concerns the production of a strain upon the application of a potential difference across the electrodes. Certain naturally occurring crystals, such as quartz and tourmaline, are piezoelectric. In these single crystals where a lattice structure is repeated at a regular manner, forming a 3D pattern throughout the material, the molecular structure does not exhibit a separation of charges; i.e., the center of the negative charge coincides with that of the positive charge.

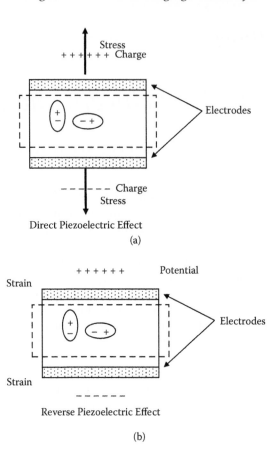

Figure 3.1 (a) Direct piezoelectric effect where a stress induces a charge separation. (b) Reverse piezoelectric effect where a potential difference across the electrodes induces a strain.

Thus, in the normal state it is neutral. Upon the application of a strain, the lattice structure is disturbed, causing a charge separation. Similarly, an applied external electric field causes the centers of the positive and negative charges to separate, resulting in a displacement, as shown in Figure 3.2. Naturally occurring piezoelectric crystals are seldom used today as transducer materials in diagnostic ultrasonic imaging because of their weak piezoelectric properties.

In a class of materials called ferroelectric materials, which are polycrystalline, the periodicity of the crystal lattices is disrupted at the so-called grain boundaries (Safari and Akdogan, 2008). Figure 3.3 shows the electron micrograph of lead zirconate titanate, $Pb(Zr, Ti)O_3$ or PZT, consisting of many grains, each of which is composed of many domains, as

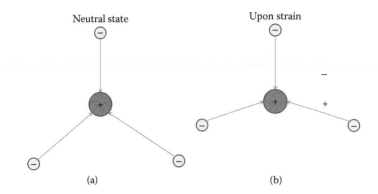

Figure 3.2 Atomic structure of a natural piezoelectric crystal (a) is distorted upon the application of external strain producing a charge separation (b).

illustrated in Figure 3.4. Ferroelectric materials have spontaneous polarization or electric dipoles as opposed to paraelectric materials, which have no spontaneous dipoles. The most popular ferroelectric material is PZT, which possesses very strong piezoelectric properties following a preparation step called poling. The physical reason that the piezoelectric phenomenon occurs in a ferroelectric material can be idealistically explained by considering that a ferroelectric material consists of many domains,

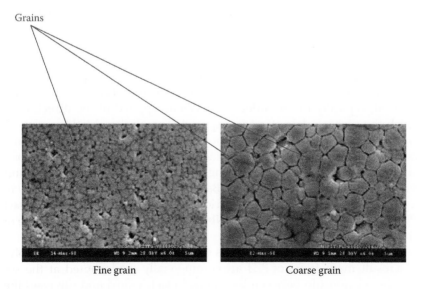

Figure 3.3 Electron micrograms of PZT materials with fine grain and coarse grain size.

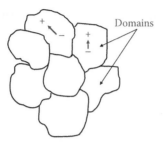

Figure 3.4 Each grain of a ferroelectric piezoelectric material consists of many domains.

each possessing innumerable electric dipoles, resulting in a net electric dipole. In the virgin state of the material, it is electrically neutral. A net dipole or polarization can be produced by poling or applying a strong electrical field in a certain direction to align the dipoles to that direction. This net polarization disappears when the temperature is raised above a material-specific level called Curie temperature, because above this temperature the directions of the net dipoles of all domains become random, thus producing no net dipole. After the material is poled, producing a net dipole for each domain, an electrical potential difference applied across a slab of piezoelectric material realigns the dipoles in the material to a preferential direction, resulting in a deformation or a change in the thickness of the slab. Conversely, a stress that causes a deformation of the material and reorientation of the dipoles induces a net charge across the electrodes.

Poling or polarization of a ferroelectric material is carried out by heating it to a temperature just above the Curie temperature of the material, and then allowing it to cool down slowly in the presence of a strong electric field, typically in the order of 20 kV/cm, applied in the direction in which the piezoelectric effect is required. The electrical field is usually applied to the material by means of two electrodes. This process aligns the dipoles along the direction of the electrical field. Poling is typically done in oil to prevent electric arcing. There are a great variety of ferroelectric materials. Barium titanate ($BaTiO_3$) was among the first that were developed. Single-crystal ferroelectric materials such as lead metaniobate ($PbNb_2O_6$) and lithium niobate ($LiNbO_3$) have also been found to possess strong piezoelectric properties.

Certain piezoelectric properties of PZT can be enhanced by doping. As a result, many types of PZT are commercially available.

The relationship between the applied electric field and the resultant polarization is material specific and, in general, has a characteristic in the form of a hysteresis loop, shown in Figure 3.5. Remanent polarization and coercive field are defined, respectively, as the value of polarization when

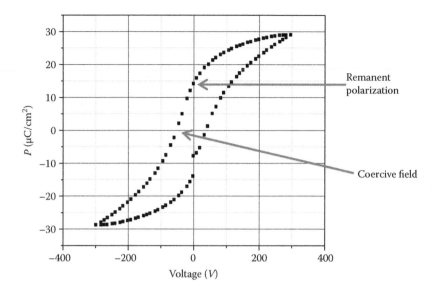

Figure 3.5 Polarization (*P*) versus electrical field or voltage (*V*) loop of a ferroelectric piezoelectric material.

the electric field = 0 or voltage = 0 after poling and the value of the electric field when there is no polarization. Remanent polarization is a measure of the piezoelectric strength of a material, whereas coercive field is a measure of the propensity of a material to depole. For both, the larger, the better.

Many ferroelectric materials have different ferroelectric states depending on the constituent composition. For instance, PZT has three different states: cubic, rhombohedral, and tetragonal, depending on the $PbTiO_3$ and $PbZrO_3$ composition, as shown in Figure 3.6. Its piezoelectric properties are the best at the morphotropic phase boundary (MPB) between the rhombohedral and tetragonal states, where the volume concentrations of $PbTiO_3$ and $PbZrO_3$ are 48 and 52%, respectively. The state of a ferroelectric material may shift from one to another at a certain temperature called phase transition temperature. Curie temperature is one of the transition temperatures. For PZT it is the transition temperature between the cubic and rhombohedral states when the $PbTiO_3$ concentration is lower than 48%. Above this temperature, the state becomes cubic and there is no net dipole. For example the Curie temperature for $BaTiO_3$ is 120°C, but there is a transition temperature at 10°C.

In order to define and better understand the physical meaning of the piezoelectric properties of a material, the constitutive equations that govern the piezoelectric effect must be examined.

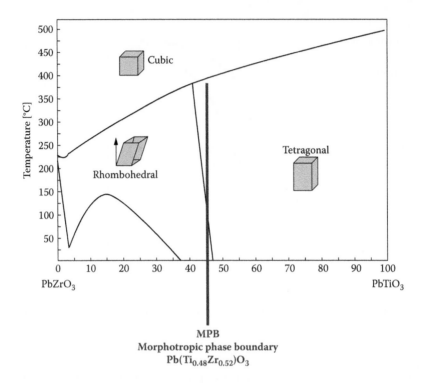

MPB
Morphotropic phase boundary
$Pb(Ti_{0.48}Zr_{0.52})O_3$

Figure 3.6 PZT has three ferroelectric states.

3.2 Piezoelectric constitutive equation

Since the piezoelectric effect involves the interaction between electric fields and the mechanical deformation, the constitutive equations relate the electric properties to mechanical properties of the material.

With no electric field, the stress and strain relationship has been described in Chapter 2, given by Equations (2.3) to (2.5). Since most materials are anisotropic, this relationship written in tensor form is given by

$$[\kappa] = [C][\varepsilon] \tag{3.1}$$

where $[\kappa]$, $[C]$, and $[\varepsilon]$ are, respectively, the stress, the elastic constant, and the strain tensor. Upon the application of an electric field, Equation (3.1) needs to be modified to include the effect of the electric field. Taking the electric field $[E]$ and the strain $[\varepsilon]$ as independent variables and the electric displacement $[D]$ and stress $[\kappa]$ as dependent variables, the piezoelectric constitutive equations are given by

$$[\kappa] = [C^E][\varepsilon] - [e][E] \tag{3.2}$$

$$[D] = [K^\varepsilon][E] + [e][\varepsilon] \tag{3.3}$$

where [e], [C^E], and [K^ε] are the piezoelectric stress constant tensor, elastic constant tensor when the electric field [E] = 0, and dielectric constant tensor when strain [ε] = 0 or clamped dielectric constant tensor. The physical meaning of [C^E] and [κ^ε] can be readily understood by setting [E] and [ε] = 0, respectively, in Equations (3.2) and (3.3). Letting [ε] = 0 in Equation (3.2),

$$[e] = -[\kappa]/[E] \tag{3.4}$$

where [e], the piezoelectric stress constant, is the resultant stress change per unit change in electric field without strain or while being clamped. It has the unit of newtons/v-m or coulombs/m^2.

The constitutive equation can be written in another form when [κ] and [E] are treated as independent variables.

$$[\varepsilon] = [d][E] + [\gamma^E][\kappa] \tag{3.5}$$

$$[D] = [K^K][E] + [d][\kappa] \tag{3.6}$$

where [K^K] is the free dielectric constant, which is the dielectric constant when there is no stress, and [d] = [ε]/[E] is the transmission or piezoelectric strain constant, representing the resultant change in strain per unit change in electric field with a unit of coulombs/newton when there is no stress. [γ^E] = [ε]/[κ] from Equation (3.5) is the compliance of the material for [E] = 0 and [γ^E] = 1/[C^E]. The relationship between [e] and [d] can be found from Equation (3.2) by setting [κ] = 0,

$$[C^E] [\varepsilon] - [e] [E] = 0$$

Therefore,

$$[e] = [C^E] [\varepsilon]/[E] = [C^E] [d]$$

If [D] and [κ] are treated as independent variables, the constitutive equations are given by

$$[E] = [\alpha^K][D] - [g][\kappa] \tag{3.7}$$

$$[\varepsilon] = [g][D] + [\gamma^D][\kappa] \tag{3.8}$$

where [g] = −[E]/[κ] is the receiving constant with a unit of volt-m/newton, representing the change in electric field per unit change in applied stress when [D] = 0; i.e., there is no current or under open circuit conditions. [γ^D] is the compliance when [D] = 0, and [α^κ] = 1/[K^κ] when [κ] = 0.

The dielectric constant [K] of a piezoelectric material depends on the extent of freedom of the material. Two values are often quoted in the literature. If the material is clamped so that it cannot move in response to an applied field or the strain is zero, the dielectric constant measured is designated as the clamped dielectric constant $[K^\varepsilon]$. If the material is free to move without restriction, the dielectric constant measured is denoted as $[K^\kappa]$, the free dielectric constant. The transmitting constant and the receiving constant are related by the following relationship (Kino, 1987):

$$[d] = [g][K^\kappa] \tag{3.9}$$

As was mentioned, these equations are in tensor form because most piezoelectric materials or crystals are anisotropic. To completely describe the piezoelectric properties of a material, 18 piezoelectric stress constants and 18 receiving constants are required. Fortunately, since these materials usually are symmetric, a smaller number of constants are actually needed. For instance, there are only five constants for quartz. For single crystals, the principal axes are defined by the crystalline axes (Cady, 1964). A plate cut with its surface perpendicular to the x-axis is called x-cut, and so forth. The x-, y-, z-directions are indicated by numbers 1, 2, 3. For polarized ferroelectric ceramics, the 3 direction is usually reserved for the polarization direction. A piezoelectric strain constant, d_{33}, represents the strain produced in the 3 direction by applying an electric field in the 3 direction, and d_{13} is the strain in the 1 direction produced by an electric field in the 3 direction when there is no external stress. Here it is important to note that the piezoelectric properties of a material depend upon boundary conditions, and therefore upon the shape of the material. For example, the piezoelectric constant of a material in the plate form is different from that in the rod form.

The capability of a piezoelectric material to convert one form of energy into another is determined by its electromechanical coupling coefficient (ECC), defined as

$$ECC = \sqrt{\frac{Stored\ Mechancial\ Energy}{Total\ Stored\ Energy}}$$

The total stored energy includes both mechanical and electrical energy. Therefore,

$$ECC^2 = \frac{Stored\ Mechanical\ Energy}{Total\ Stored\ Eenergy}$$

It should be noted that this quantity is not the efficiency of the transducer. If the transducer is lossless, its efficiency is 100%, but the

Table 3.1 Properties of Important Piezoelectric Materials

Property	PVDF	Quartz (X-Cut)	PZT-5H	Lead Niobate
d_{33} (10^{-12} c/n)	15	2.31	583	100
g_{33} (10^{-2} v-m/n)	14	5.78	191	430
ECC_t	0.11	0.14	0.55	0.34
K^κ (10^{-11} F/m)	9.7	3.98	3010	3054
c (m/s)	2070	5740	3970	3100
ρ (kg/m^3)	1760	2650	7450	5900
Curie temp (°C)	100	573	190	500

ρ *and c denote density and sound speed, respectively.*

electromechanical coupling coefficient is not necessarily 100% because some of the energy is stored as mechanical energy and the rest is stored dielectrically in the form of electrical potential energy. Since only the stored mechanical energy is useful, the electromechanical coupling coefficient is a measure of the performance of a material as a transducer. The piezoelectric constants for a few important piezoelectric materials are listed in Table 3.1.

There are a few important material geometries that are frequently encountered in ultrasonic imaging. These are shown in Figure 3.7 using the effect of geometry on an electromechanical coupling coefficient as an example. For a disc of PZT-5H with the diameter much larger than the thickness (c), the thickness mode electromechanical coupling coefficient

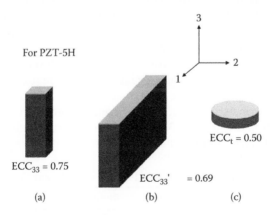

Figure 3.7 The effect of a piezoelectric material affects its piezoelectric properties. This is illustrated by way of the electrical mechanical coupling coefficient. (a) A tall element of square cross section frequently seen in composite materials. (b) A tall element frequently seen in linear arrays. (c) A circular disc frequently seen in single-element transducers.

ECC$_t$ is used. For a long tall element with the sides of the square cross section much smaller than the thickness (a) and a tall element with rectangular cross section (b), the electromechanical coupling coefficients are denoted as ECC$_{33}$ and ECC$_{33}$', respectively. The geometry shown in Figure 3.7(b) is the most important in that it is often used in linear arrays. It is interesting to note that the electromechanical coupling coefficient is highest in the bar mode shown in (a), attributable to the fact that more energy is irradiated in the long-axis direction because the bar is surrounded by air, which has a much lower acoustic impedance than PZT. The effect of material shape on other measured piezoelectric properties can be found in Table 3.2. There is an additional definition for ECC, the planar ECC or ECC$_p$, which is defined as the strain or displacement generated in the 1 or 2 direction of a thin disc for an electric field applied in the 3 direction.

Ferroelectric ceramics are often classified as soft or hard by their rigidity. In general, soft ceramics have larger piezoelectric constants, dielectric constants, ECC, and loss, but poorer linearity. They are also easier to pole.

In addition to PZT, piezoelectric polymers have also been found to be useful in a number of applications (Brown, 2000). One of these polymers is polyvinylidence difluoride (PVDF), which is semicrystalline. After processes like polymerization, stretching, and poling, a thin sheet of PVDF with a thickness in the order of 6 to 50 µm can be used as a transducer material. The advantages of this material are that it is wideband, flexible, and inexpensive. The disadvantages are that it has a very low transmitting constant, its dielectric loss is large, and the dielectric constant is low. Although PVDF is not an ideal transmitting material, it does possess a fairly high receiving constant. Miniature PVDF hydrophones are commercially available. P(VDF-TrFE) co-polymers have been shown to have a higher electromechanical coupling coefficient.

One of the most promising frontiers in transducer technology is the development of piezoelectric composite materials (Smith, 1989). Innovation in fabrication technology has allowed the preparation of PZT polymer 1-3 composites for applications in the 1 to 7.5 MHz range. These 1-3 composites, consisting of small PZT rods embedded in a low-density polymer, illustrated in Figure 3.8, where the dark and light regions indicate the piezoelectric ceramic phase and the polymer phase, respectively,

Table 3.2 Material Properties of PZT-5H of Different Geometries

Property	Bar mode	Plate mode	Element mode
Velocity (m/s)	3850	4580	4000
Acoustic impedance (Mrayl)	28.9	34.3	30.0
Electromechanical coupling coefficient	0.75	0.51	0.73

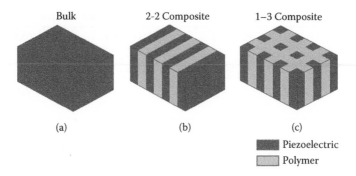

Figure 3.8 Configurations of piezoelectric composites: (a) Bulk, (b) 2-2 composites, and (c) 1-3 composites.

have been used for low-frequency underwater applications for many years. The notation 1-3, 2-2, etc., has been coined by Newnham et al. (1978). A notation of 1-3 means that one phase of the composite is connected only in one direction, whereas the second phase is connected in all three directions. A notation of 2-2 means that both phases are connected in two directions, as illustrated in Figure 3.8. These composites, typically in volume concentration of 20 to 70% PZT, have a lower acoustic impedance (4 to 25 MRayl) than conventional PZT (34 MRayl), which better matches the acoustic impedance of human skin. The composite material can be made flexible with a free dielectric constant, K^κ, from $44 \cdot 10^{-11}$ to $2213 \cdot 10^{-11}$ F/m, and with an ECC_t higher than that of PZT. The higher coupling coefficient and better impedance matching can lead to higher transducer sensitivity and improved image resolution. An electron micrograph of a 2-2 composite is shown in Figure 3.9 with 28 µm PZT-5H piezoelectric ceramics and 5 µm polymer filler. In designing composites, care must be taken to avoid spurious lateral resonance modes. The height of a square pillar should be

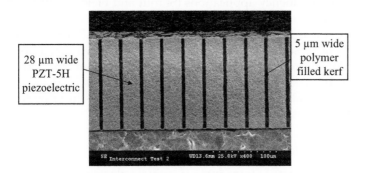

Figure 3.9 An electron micrograph of a 2-2 composite consisting of PZT-5H piezoelectrics separated by polymer.

Table 3.3 Piezoelectric Properties of Single-Crystal Piezoelectric Materials

Property	PZN-PT	PMN-PT	PIN-PMN-PT
ECC_{33}	0.93	0.94	0.94
Tc, °C	140	155	160
K^ε	294	800	700
Z, MRayl	26	30	30

much larger than the width of the sides and the width of the kerf, which is the gap among the pillars. The pillar and the kerf width should all be much smaller than the wavelength. The lateral resonance modes are also determined by the filler material, which must be carefully chosen. Epo-Tech 301-2 is a popular filler material that has a longitudinal velocity of 2650 m/s, a shear velocity of 1230 m/s, and a density of 1150 kg/m^3. It also has fairly large attenuation coefficients for longitudinal (9.5 dB/mm at 30 MHz) and shear (3.6 dB/mm at 30 MHz) waves.

One of the problems associated with composite materials is the higher fabrication cost. Typical fabrication approaches include (1) dice and fill where PZT is first diced and subsequently the gaps are filled with a polymer, and (2) injection molding. The performances of composite annular and linear arrays with frequencies from 3 to 7.5 MHz have been found to be superior to those of similar PZT devices. A substantial number of commercial high-performance arrays are made from composites.

Conventional PZT has a grain size in the order of 3 to 5 μm, which is not particularly suited for high-frequency applications. Fine-grain PZT and single-crystal ferroelectric materials like $Pb(Zn_{1/3}Nb_{2/3})O_3$-$PbTiO_3$ (PZN-PT), $Pb(Mg_{1/3}Nb_{2/3})O_3$-$PbTiO_3$ (PMN-PT), and $Pb(In_{1/2}Nb_{1/2})$-$Pb(Mg_{1/3}Nb_{2/3})O_3$-$PbTiO_3$ (PIN-PMN-PT), which have been shown to have a higher dielectric constant and electromechanical coupling coefficient than conventional PZT, are potentially promising piezoelectric materials for high-frequency applications (Shrout and Fielding, 1990; Zipparo et al., 1997; Tian et al., 2007). These materials possess extremely high ECC. Their ECC_{33} was found to be as high as 0.9. Table 3.3 lists piezoelectric properties of these single-crystal materials. It is known that a number of commercial clinical scanner probes at frequencies from 3 to 7 MHz now are made from single-crystal piezoelectric materials, and they exhibit superior bandwidth and sensitivity, measures of transducer performance that will be discussed below.

3.3 Ultrasonic transducers

The simplest ultrasonic transducer is a single-element piston transducer shown in Figure 3.10, where (a) and (b) show, respectively, a photo and the internal construction of a single-element ultrasonic transducer. The most

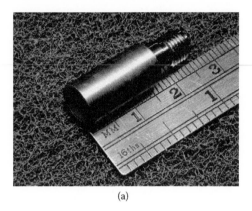

(a)

Lithium Niobate Transducers

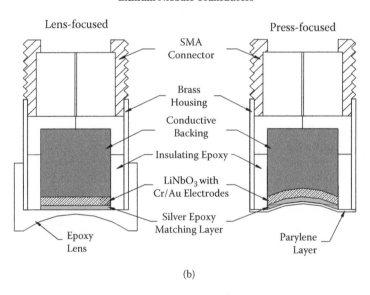

(b)

Figure 3.10 (a) Photo and (b) detailed construction of two single-element ultrasonic transducers with one or two matching layers and the backing material. The transducer on the left has a lens, whereas the one on the right is self-focused.

important component of such a device is the piezoelectric element. A number of factors are involved in choosing a proper piezoelectric material for transmitting or receiving the ultrasonic wave. They include stability, piezoelectric properties, and the strength of the material. The surfaces of the element are electroded with fired-on silver or sputtered chrome-gold. The outside electrode is usually grounded to protect the patients from electrical shock. The housing is metallic or plastic. An acoustic isolating

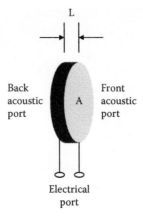

L

Back
acoustic
port

A

Front
acoustic
port

Electrical
port

Figure 3.11 A piezoceramic disc can be treated as an electromechanical device with two acoustic ports representing the front and rear interfaces between the ceramic and the surrounding media and an electrical port.

material is placed between the piezoelectric element and the housing to prevent ringing of the housing that follows the vibration of the piezoelectric element itself.

By considering the two surfaces of the piezoelectric element as two independent vibrators, as illustrated in Figure 3.11, one can easily see that the resonant frequencies for such a transducer are given by

$$f_o = \frac{nc_p}{2L} \tag{3.10}$$

with the lowest resonant frequency being $n = 1$, where c_p is the acoustic wave velocity in the transducer material, L is the thickness of the piezoelectric material, and n is an odd integer. In other words, resonance occurs when L is equal to odd multiples of one-half wavelength, or

$$L = n\frac{\lambda_p}{2} \tag{3.11}$$

where λ_p is the wavelength in the piezoelectric material.

The transducer can be treated as a three-port network, as shown in Figure 3.12, two being mechanical ports representing the front and back surfaces of the piezoelectric crystal and one being an electrical port representing the electrical connection of the piezoelectric material to the electrical generator (Kino, 1987). Various sophisticated one-dimensional (1D) circuit models exist to model the behavior of the transducer. The most well known are the Mason model, the Redwood

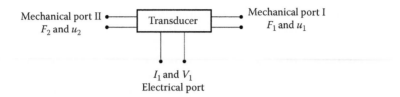

Figure 3.12 A system model for a single-element transducer.

model, and the KLM model. Commercial software based on these models is available.

The Mason model can be derived by considering the three-port configuration shown in Figure 3.13 for a circular disc with area A and thickness L, where I, V, F, and u denote current, voltage, force, and medium velocity, respectively.

Using the transmission line theory, the constitutive equations relating mechanical properties to electrical properties, and boundary conditions that u and F must be continuous across interfaces, the following simultaneous equations can be obtained:

$$
\begin{bmatrix} F_1 \\ F_2 \\ V_3 \end{bmatrix} = -j \begin{bmatrix} Z_c \cot k_p L & Z_c \cos ec k_p L & \dfrac{e}{\omega K^\varepsilon} \\ Z_c \cos ec k_p L & Z_c \cot k_p L & \dfrac{e}{\omega K^\varepsilon} \\ \dfrac{e}{\omega K^\varepsilon} & \dfrac{e}{\omega K^\varepsilon} & \dfrac{1}{\omega C_0} \end{bmatrix} \begin{bmatrix} u_1 \\ u_2 \\ I_3 \end{bmatrix} \qquad (3.12)
$$

where $Z_c = Z_0 A$ is called the radiation impedance and Z_0 is the acoustic impedance of the piezoelectric element, e is the piezoelectric stress constant, k_p is the wave number in the piezoelectric material, and $C_0 = K_\varepsilon (A/L)$, the

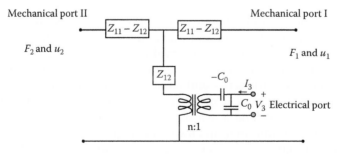

Figure 3.13 The Mason model or equivalent circuit for a single-element transducer.

clamped capacitance. These simultaneous equations can be represented by an electrical equivalent network, shown in Figure 3.8, where $Z_{11} = -jZ_c\cot(k_pL)$, $Z_{12} = -jZ_c\text{cosec}(k_pL)$, $Z_{11} - Z_{12} = jZ_c\tan(k_pL/2)$, and $n = e(A/L)$.

Assuming that the loading media have acoustic impedances Z_1 and Z_2, respectively, at ports I and II, the input electrical impedance Z_3 of the transducer at the electrical port can be readily calculated using this equivalent network.

$$Z_3 = \frac{V_3}{I_3} = \frac{1}{j\omega C_0}\left\{1 + ECC_t^2 \frac{j(Z_1 + Z_2)Z_c \sin k_pL - 2Z_c^2(1 - \cos k_pL)}{[(Z_c^2 + Z_1Z_2)\sin k_pL - j(Z_1 + Z_2)Z_c \cos k_pL]k_pL}\right\}$$

(3.13)

For the special case where Z_1 and $Z_2 = 0$, this means a disc loaded by air on both sides. Z_3 becomes

$$Z_3 = \frac{1}{j\omega C_0} + Z_a$$
(3.14)

where Z_a is given by

$$Z_a = -\frac{ECC_t^2}{j\omega C_0}\frac{\tan(k_pL/2)}{k_pL/2}$$
(3.15)

Equation (3.14) can be represented by an equivalent network consisting of an impedance Z_a in series with a capacitor C_0. It can be shown easily that $Z_a \rightarrow -ECC_t^2/(j\omega C_0)$ when $\omega \rightarrow 0$. Therefore, at low frequencies a circular disc resonating in air basically behaves like a free capacitor $C_0^\kappa = Z_a + C_0 = K^\kappa(A/L)$. As $\omega \rightarrow \infty$, Equation (3.14) yields $Z_3 \rightarrow 1/(j\omega C_0)$. It behaves like a clamped capacitor, $C_0 = K^\varepsilon(A/L)$. This phenomenon has been used as a method for measuring K^ε and K^κ of a piezoelectric material.

A more careful examination of Equation (3.13) shows that the input impedance has a minimum and maximum as a function of frequency for a transducer irradiating into a medium with acoustic impedance Z_1 with a backing medium of acoustic impedance Z_2. These frequencies are called, respectively, the series and parallel resonant frequencies. At these frequencies the transducer can be represented by two-port networks consisting of a capacitor and a resistor. At series resonance or simply resonance, $\omega = \omega_r$, Z_3 is minimal, and the phase angle changes from $-90°$ to $90°$. At parallel or antiresonance, $\omega = \omega_a$, Z_3 is maximal, and the phase angle changes from $90°$ to $-90°$. These two networks are shown in Figure 3.14(a)

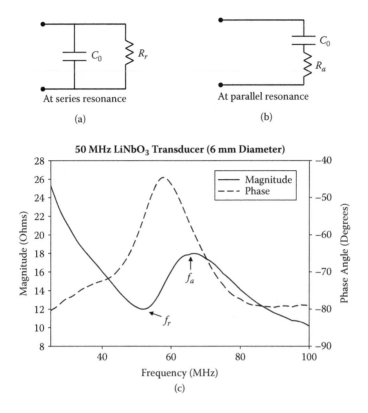

Figure 3.14 Equivalent electrical network for a single-element transducer near resonance: (a) at series resonance and (b) at parallel resonance. (c) The magnitude and phase of the input electrical impedance of a circular disc resonating in air as a function of frequency.

and (b), where R_a and R_r are, respectively, the radiation resistances at parallel and series resonances and are given by

$$R_a = \frac{4ECC_t^2 Z_c}{\pi \omega_a C_0 (Z_1 + Z_2)} \tag{3.16}$$

$$R_r = \frac{\pi (Z_1 + Z_2)}{4ECC_t^2 \omega_r C_0 Z_c} \tag{3.17}$$

A plot of the magnitude and phase of a circular disc resonating in air as a function of frequency is shown in Figure 3.14(c), where the resonance and antiresonance frequencies and the change in phase near these frequencies are clearly seen. A more popular 1D transducer mode is the KLM model, which is shown in Figure 3.15. This model divides a piezoelectric

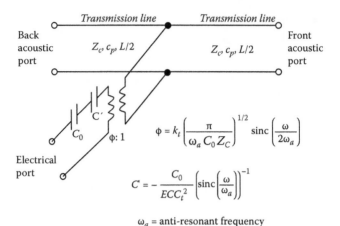

$$\phi = k_t \left(\frac{\pi}{\omega_a C_0 Z_C} \right)^{1/2} \text{sinc} \left(\frac{\omega}{2\omega_a} \right)$$

$$C' = -\frac{C_0}{ECC_t^2} \left[\text{sinc} \left(\frac{\omega}{\omega_a} \right) \right]^{-1}$$

ω_a = anti-resonant frequency

Figure 3.15 The KLM model for a single-element transducer.

element into two halves, each represented by a transmission line. It is more physically intuitive. The effects of matching layers and backing material can be readily included.

A typical response for a PZT-5A single-element transducer of 1 cm diameter, 5.5 MHz resonant frequency, loaded by water, and air backed, obtained with the KLM model, is given in Figure 3.16. Both the pulse-echo

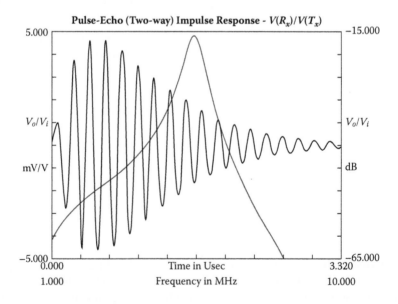

Figure 3.16 The pulse-echo waveform and its spectrum of a single-element transducer with no matching and backing obtained by the KLM model.

waveform and the echo spectrum are shown. The vertical scale is the ratio of output voltage/input voltage in mv/v. A Q factor can be defined for the transducer as

$$Q = f_o/(f_2 - f_1) \tag{3.18}$$

where f_o is the resonant frequency and f_2 and f_1 are the frequencies at which the amplitude drops to −3 or −6 dB relative to the maximum. The difference, $f_2 - f_1$, is referred to as the bandwidth of the transducer. Two Q factors, electrical Q and mechanical Q, have been used to describe ultrasonic transducers since, after all, they are electromechanical devices. In applications where maximal output is needed and bandwidth requirement is not crucial, as in a continuous-wave ultrasonic Doppler flowmeter, the Q of the transducer should be large, whereas in pulse-echo imaging devices, the Q should be small, in the order of 1 to 2. To adjust the Q or bandwidth of a transducer, either electrical matching, which optimizes electrical Q, or mechanical matching, which optimizes mechanical Q, can be used.

3.3.1 Mechanical matching

When a transducer is excited by an electrical source, it rings at its natural resonant frequency. For continuous-wave application, the transducers are air backed, allowing as much energy irradiated into the forward medium (like water, which has higher acoustic impedance than air), as possible. Due to the mismatch in acoustic impedance between the air and the piezoelectric material, acoustic energy at this interface is reflected into the forward direction. Thus, very little energy is lost out of the back port. The drawback is that this mismatch, which produces the so-called ringing effect for pulse-echo applications, is very undesirable because it lengthens the pulse duration. As will be discussed later, the pulse duration affects the capability of an imaging system for resolving small objects.

Absorptive backing materials with acoustic impedance similar to that of the piezoelectric material can be used to damp out the ringing or to increase bandwidth. The backing material should not only absorb part of the energy from the vibration of the back face, but also minimize the mismatch in acoustic impedance. It absorbs as much as possible the energy that enters it. It must be noted that suppression of ringing or shortening of pulse duration is achieved by sacrificing sensitivity, because a large portion of the energy is absorbed by the backing material. Various types of backing materials, including tungsten-loaded epoxy and silver-loaded epoxy, have been used with good success. Several backing materials are listed in Table 3.4.

The performance of a transducer can also be improved with acoustic matching layers mounted in the front. It can be easily shown that for a

Table 3.4 Acoustic Properties of Transducer Materials

Matching layers	Acoustic impedance (MRayl)	Sound velocity (mm/μs)	Reference
Ceramic-loaded epoxy	2.8–11.3	1.5–3.9	Selfridge, 1985
Glass	10.1–16.0	4.5–5.66	Selfridge, 1985
Parylene	2.83 (Parylene C)	2.20	Thiagarajan et al., 1991
Si/RTV composite	Tapered from 1.5 to 12 through thickness (experimental)	1.0–8.0 (theoretical)	Sayers and Tait, 1984
Backing Material			
Tungsten-loaded epoxy	6–36	1.5–3.5	Kino, 1987
Brass (70% Cu, 30% Zn)	40.6	4.70	Selfridge, 1985
Carbon, pyrolytic	7.31	3.31	Selfridge, 1985
Air	0.00043	0.334	Selfridge, 1985
Lens Material			
RTV rubber	0.99–1.46	0.96–1.16	Selfridge, 1985
Polyurethane	1.38–2.36	1.33–2.09	Selfridge, 1985
Silicone rubber (Sylgard)	1.03	1.05	Kino, 1987
Composite Fillers			
RTV	0.99–1.46	0.96–1.16	Kino, 1987
Epoxy	2.8–6.0	2.7	Gururaja et al., 1985
Polyurethane (Tetrad)	1.26	2.43	Gururaja et al., 1985
Polyurethane (MSI solid 80)	1.14	2.27	Gururaja et al., 1985
Polymer/microballoon	0.5	2.02	Shung and Zipparo, 1996

monochromatic plane wave, 100% transmission occurs for a layer of material of $\lambda_m/4$ thickness and acoustic impedance Z_m, where λ_m is the wavelength in the matching layer material (Kinsler and Frey, 2000).

$$Z_m = (Z_p Z_l)^{1/2} \tag{3.19}$$

In Equation (3.19), Z_p and Z_l are, respectively, the acoustic impedances of the piezoelectric element and the loading medium.

For wideband transducers, however, Desilets et al. (1978) showed that for a single matching layer, Equation (3.19) should be modified to

$$Z_m = (Z_p Z_1^2)^{1/3} \tag{3.20}$$

and for two matching layers, the acoustic impedances of the two layers should be, respectively,

$$Z_{m1} = (Z_p^4 Z_1^3)^{1/7} \tag{3.21}$$

$$Z_{m2} = (Z_p Z_1^6)^{1/7} \tag{3.22}$$

State-of-the-art transducers and arrays that use composites can achieve a bandwidth better than 70% merely with front matching and light backing without losing much sensitivity. The reason for this is that optimal matching allows energy to be transmitted into the forward direction and reduces ringing resulting from reverberation of pulses, thus widening the bandwidth. Some of the materials that have been used for matching layers and filler materials in composites are tabulated in Table 3.4.

3.3.2 Electrical matching

Maximizing energy transmission or bandwidth can also be achieved by matching the electrical characteristics of the transducer to the electrical source and amplifier. Circuit components may be placed between the transducer and external electrical devices (Desilets et al., 1978; Goldberg and Smith, 1994). Consider the equivalent circuit for a transducer at series resonance shown in Figure 3.14(a). For maximal power transmission, the transducer input impedance should be real and the input resistance should match that of the source. To tune out the clamped capacitance, a shunt inductor of the value $1/(\omega_r^2 C_0)$ may be used. A shunt inductor of the value $1/(\omega_a^2 C_0) + R_a^2 C_0$ can be used for the circuit at parallel resonance, shown in Figure 3.14(b). A transformer may be used to match the resistance.

The substantial improvement in transducer performance by including acoustic matching, backing, and electrical tuning in the design of a 5.1 MHz PZT-5A transducer is demonstrated in Figure 3.17, where a 72% bandwidth and a much improved sensitivity are seen.

3.4 Characterization of piezoelectric materials

3.4.1 Dielectric constant

The dielectric constant K of a piezoelectric material can be measured with a circular disc prepared from the piezoelectric material and fixed in air with a spring clip fixture, as shown in Figure 3.18. The electrical

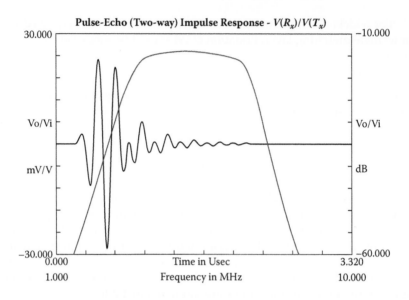

Figure 3.17 The performance of the transducer is improved by matching and backing.

impedance Z_3 is measured with an impedance analyzer. K is related to Z_3 by the following equation:

$$K = \frac{L}{\omega |Z_3| A} \qquad (3.23)$$

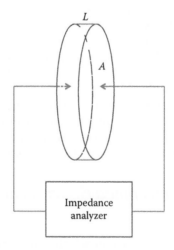

Figure 3.18 Experimental arrangement for measuring dielectric constant of a piezoelectric material.

where L and A are the thickness and area of the disc. Electrical impedances measured at lower and higher frequencies relative to the resonant
frequency of the transducer yield, respectively, the free and clamped
dielectric constants of the piezoelectric material.

3.4.2 Dielectric loss tangent

If the dielectric loss in a piezoelectric material is small, and this is the case
in the low MHz range, it may be ignored. The loss, however, increases as
the frequency increases. To take the loss into consideration, the dielectric
constant is made complex, i.e., $K = K' + jK''$, where K'' denotes the loss
term. The loss tangent defined as K''/K' is related to the measured electrical impedance of a disc, shown in Figure 3.18, by

$$\tan\delta_e = \frac{K''}{K'} = \frac{1}{\tan\theta}$$

where θ is the phase angle of the complex input electrical impedance Z_3. It
follows from the preceding sections on dielectric constants that there are two
loss tangents: clamped and free loss tangents. This relationship can be found
by looking at the input electrical impedance of a disc suspended in air:

$$Z_3 = \frac{1}{j\omega C} = \frac{1}{j\omega K \dfrac{A}{L}} = -j\frac{L}{\omega A}\frac{1}{K' + jK''} = \frac{-L}{\omega A\left(K'^2 + K''^2\right)}(K'' + jK')$$

where the phase angle $\theta = \tan^{-1}(K'/K'')$ or $\tan\theta = K'/K'' = 1/\tan\delta_e$. Therefore,
the loss tangents of a piezoelectric material can be readily determined by
measuring the complex input electrical impedance to a disc in air. The
ratio of imaginary and real parts of Z_3 yields $\tan\theta$.

3.4.3 Electromechanical coupling coefficient

To measure the thickness mode electromechanical coupling coefficient
ECC_t of a piezoelectric material, a circular disc is prepared and arranged
as shown in Figure 3.18. The input electrical impedance of the disc Z_3
near resonance is given by Equation (3.14). At antiresonance, $Z_3 \to \infty$
and $k_p L/2 = (\omega_a L)/(2c_p) = \pi/2$. Therefore, $\omega_a = (\pi c_p)/L$, and at resonance,
$\tan(k_p L/2) = \tan[(\omega_r L)/(2c_p)] = \tan\dfrac{\pi\omega_r}{2\frac{\pi c_p}{L}} = \tan\dfrac{\pi\omega_r}{2\omega_a}$ and $Z_3 \to 0$. As a result,

$$ECC_t^2 \frac{\tan\dfrac{\pi\omega_r}{2\omega_a}}{\dfrac{\pi\omega_r}{2\omega_a}} = 1$$

Rearranging this equation, it can be found that

$$ECC_t^2 = \frac{\dfrac{\pi f_r}{2 f_a}}{\tan \dfrac{\pi f_r}{2 f_a}} \tag{3.24}$$

This equation indicates that ECC_t can be readily measured by determining the resonant and antiresonant frequencies from the measured Z_3. If $(ECC_t)^2$ is <0.5, it can be estimated from the following equation within 15% (Kino, 1987):

$$ECC_t = \frac{\pi}{2\sqrt{2}} \sqrt{1 - \left(\frac{f_r}{f_a}\right)^2}$$

Equation (3.24) can be easily converted to the IEEE standards (ASNE/ IEEE, 1987).

$$ECC_t^2 = \frac{\pi f_r}{2 f_a} \tan \frac{\pi (f_a - f_r)}{2 f_a}$$

Previous discussions pertain to lossless or low-loss piezoelectric materials. As the frequency is increased, the losses can no longer be ignored and must be taken into consideration in the estimation of ECC. Methods have been developed to do so (Foster et al., 1991; Zipparo et al., 1997). One such method (Foster et al., 1991) utilized the KLM model of a circular disc surrounded by air. The results found that the ECC of piezoelectric materials drops as frequency is increased and suggested that this degradation in ECC might be remedied if the grain size is reduced.

3.4.4 Mechanical quality factor Q_m

The mechanical quality factor of a piezoelectric material is defined as (Ristic, 1983)

$$Q_m = \frac{\omega(average\ stored\ energy)}{dissipated\ energy} = \frac{\omega}{2 c_p \alpha_p}$$

Since $f\lambda_p = c_p$, it can be shown that $Q_m = \pi/\alpha_p \lambda_p$, where α_p is the attenuation coefficient in the piezoelectric material. It is inversely proportional to the mechanical energy loss in one wavelength. A material with high Q_m means that it has a smaller mechanical loss. It can be measured from a

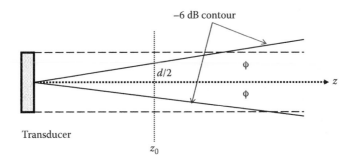

Figure 3.19 Mechanism used by a d_{33} meter to measure d_{33}.

measurement of the ultrasonic attenuation coefficient of the piezoelectric material or estimated from the modified KLM model that includes acoustic attenuation by measuring the input electrical impedance of a circular disc prepared from this material surrounded by air (Foster et al., 1991; Zipparo et al., 1997).

3.4.5 Piezoelectric strain or transmission constant d_{33}

Commercial devices called d_{33} meters are available for measuring this constant. In these devices a force is applied in the order of a few newtons to the sample held between two round-shaped holders, as shown in Figure 3.19, and the charge generated on the surface of the sample is measured. The constant d_{33} is found from the ratio of charge/force in coulombs/newton.

Table 3.1 lists the constants in a few important piezoelectric materials.

3.5 Transducer beam characteristics

The beam characteristics produced by an ultrasonic transducer are far from ideal. They deviate significantly in many ways from an ideal parallel beam with a uniform intensity profile, as illustrated in Figure 3.20, which shows the most ideal case, a pencil-like beam (a) or a beam that has uniform intensity within the beam boundary and zero intensity elsewhere (b). Unfortunately a beam produced by an ultrasonic transducer is far from it. The intensity is the highest at the center and decreases as a function of the distance from the center, as in (c). It is possible to calculate the beam profile utilizing Huygens' principle (Kinsler and Frey, 2000), which states that the resultant wavefront generated by a source of finite aperture can be obtained by considering the source to be composed of an infinite number of point sources, each emitting a spherical wave. The summation of the spherical wavelets generated by all point sources on the transducer surface at a certain point yields the field at that point.

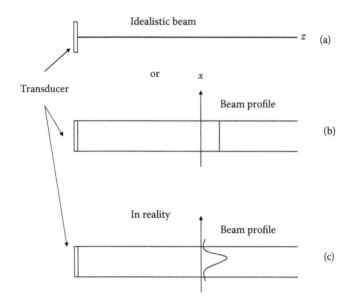

Figure 3.20 An ultrasonic beam is far from ideal. (a) idealistic beam, (b) beam profile, and (c) beam profile in reality.

Referring to Figure 3.21(a), the pressure at (r,φ,t) is given by the Rayleigh integral (Kinsler and Frey, 2000):

$$p(r,\varphi,t) = \frac{jk\rho c}{2\pi} \int_0^a \frac{u(x)e^{j(\omega t - kr')}}{r'} ds \tag{3.25}$$

where k is the wave number = $2\pi/\lambda$, ρ is the density in the propagating medium, c is the sound velocity in the propagating medium, $u(x)$ is the medium velocity on the surface of the piston transducer of radius a, $r' = \sqrt{r^2 + \sigma^2}$, S is the surface of the circular aperture = $\pi\sigma^2$, and ds is the incremental surface area = $2\pi\sigma d\sigma$. For uniform excitation shown in Figure 3.21(b), Equation (3.25) can be reduced to

$$p(r,\varphi,t) = \frac{jk\rho c}{2\pi} u_0 e^{j\omega t} \int_0^a \frac{e^{-jkr'}}{r'} 2\pi\sigma d\sigma \tag{3.26}$$

Substituting $r' = \sqrt{r^2 + \sigma^2}$ into Equation (3.26), making use of the relationship below, and carrying out the integration,

$$\frac{\sigma e^{-jk\sqrt{r^2+\sigma^2}}}{\sqrt{r^2+\sigma^2}} d\sigma = -d\frac{e^{-jk\sqrt{r^2+\sigma^2}}}{jk}$$

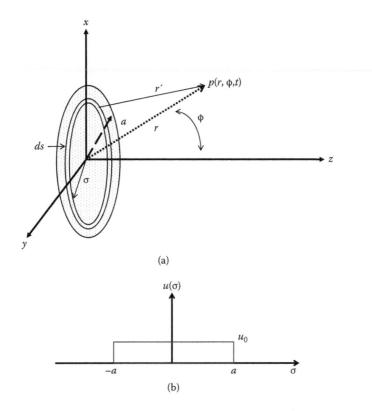

(a)

(b)

Figure 3.21 (a) Coordinate system for depicting the pressure or intensity distribution of a disc piston transducer. (b) A disc is uniform excited with a medium velocity, u_0.

$p(r,\varphi,t)$ can be found to be

$$p(r,\varphi,t) = \rho c u_0 e^{j(\omega t - kr)}(1 - e^{-jk\sqrt{r^2+a^2}-r})$$ (3.27)

To determine the pressure distribution along the z-axis or axial direction, by substituting $r = z$ into Equation (3.27), this equation becomes

$$p(z,0,t) = \rho c u_0 e^{j(\omega t - kz)}(1 - e^{-jk\sqrt{z^2+a^2}-z})$$ (3.28)

The term magnitude of the $1 - e^{-jk\sqrt{z^2+a^2}-z}$ can be further simplified to $2\sin\frac{k\sqrt{z^2+a^2}-z}{2}$. In the far field of the transducer, $z \gg a$, making use of the approximation $\sqrt{1+x} \approx 1 + \frac{1}{2}x$, it can be readily shown that $\frac{k\sqrt{z^2+a^2}-z}{2} \approx ka^2/(4z)$. When $ka^2/(4z) = n\pi/2$, $\sin\frac{k\sqrt{z^2+a^2}-z}{2} = 1$ and p is at a maximum, i.e., $p_{max} = \rho c u_0$.

At $n = 1$, p is at the last maximum and $z = z_0 = a^2/\lambda$. This distance is called the far-field near-field transition point. The regions where $z < z_0$ and $z > z_0$ are called, respectively, near field or Fresnel zone and far field or Fraunhoffer zone. In the far field, making the assumption $\sin x \approx x$ and removing the time dependence from Equation (3.28), the magnitude of the pressure along the axis becomes

$$|p(z)| = 2\rho c u_0 \left[\frac{kz}{2} \left(\sqrt{1 + \frac{a^2}{z^2}} - 1 \right) \right] = \rho c u_0 \frac{ka^2}{2z}$$

At $z = \pi a^2/\lambda$, called Rayleigh distance, $|p(z)| = (1/2) p_{max}$. This equation also shows that in the far field of a transducer, starting from

$$z_0 = a^2/\lambda \tag{3.29}$$

the pressure and intensity decrease as functions of $1/z$ and $1/z^2$, respectively. Figure 3.22 shows the continuous-wave (a) and pulsed (b) axial intensity profiles of a 5 MHz, 1 cm diameter unfocused circular transducer with natural focus at 2.9 cm.

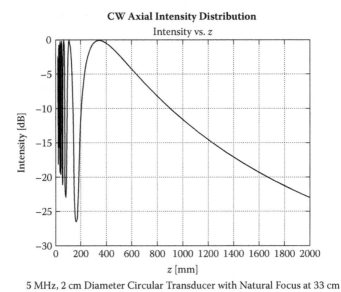

CW Axial Intensity Distribution

5 MHz, 2 cm Diameter Circular Transducer with Natural Focus at 33 cm

(a)

Figure 3.22 Axial pressure profile as a function of distance (z) for a 5 MHz piston transducer of 1 cm diameter for (a) continuous wave (CW) and (b) pulsed excitation.

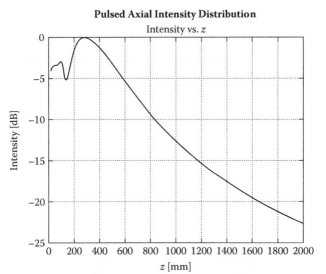

5 MHz, 2 cm Diameter Circular Transducer with Natural Focus at 33 cm

(b)

Figure 3.22 *(Continued)* Axial pressure profile as a function of distance (z) for a 5 MHz piston transducer of 1 cm diameter for (a) continuous wave (CW) and (b) pulsed excitation.

3.5.1 Lateral beam profiles

In the far field, the angular radiation pattern can be found from the Rayleigh integral as well. For a circular aperture of radius a, it is given by

$$H_c(\varphi) = H_c(\varphi = 0)\frac{2J_1(ka\sin\varphi)}{ka\sin\varphi} \qquad (3.30)$$

where J_1 is the Bessel function of the first kind of order 1. Equation (3.30) is plotted in Figure 3.23(a), which shows the angular intensity radiation pattern in the far field of a circular ultrasonic transducer consisting of a main lobe and several side lobes. The number of side lobes and their magnitude relative to that of the main lobe depend on the ratio of transducer aperture size to wavelength and the shape of the piezoelectric element. The first zero occurs at

$$\sin\varphi = 0.61 \; (\lambda/a) \qquad (3.31)$$

The first side lobe level (SSL) is –17.5 dB below the main lobe and occurs at $\varphi = \sin^{-1}(0.8\lambda/a)$. As the ratio of the aperture size to wavelength

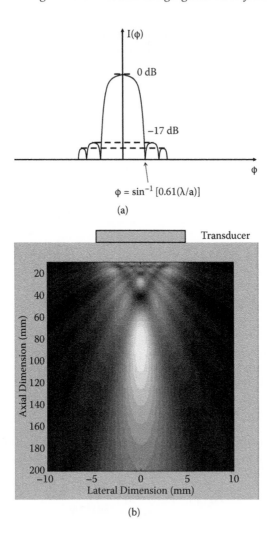

Figure 3.23 (a) Angular radiation pattern of a disc piston transducer. (b) A gray-scale representation of the acoustic field produced by a circular piston transducer of 1 cm diameter at 5 MHz.

becomes larger, ϕ decreases or the beam becomes sharper, accompanied by an increase in the number of side lobes. Side lobes are very undesirable in ultrasonic imaging because they produce spurious signals, resulting in artifacts in the image and a reduction in contrast resolution. Therefore, to have a sharper beam by increasing the ratio of transducer aperture size to wavelength, more side lobes are introduced and z_0 is shifted farther away from the transducer. Consequently, for a particular application, a compromise has to be reached or a lens may be used to shift the focal point closer

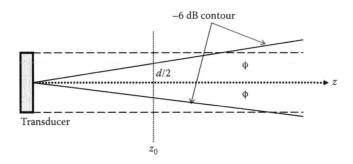

Figure 3.24 Idealistic representation of the beam behavior of a single-element piston transducer.

to the transducer. A gray-scale representation of the acoustic field produced by a circular piston transducer of 1 cm diameter at 5 MHz is shown in Figure 3.23(b), where $z_0 = 8.1$ cm. Here the brightness is proportional to pressure amplitude.

The transverse profile in the near field is extremely complex and not well defined. As z becomes greater than z_0, the beam starts to diverge, illustrated in Figure 3.24, which is an idealistic representation of the beam behavior of a circular piston transducer. In the near field it behaves more or less like a parallel beam and starts to diverge at z_0 at an angle of ϕ. In the very far field, the transducer behaves like a point source irradiating energy into a cone confined to an angle defined by 2ϕ. The beam boundary is represented by the −3 or −6 dB contour. At z_0 the beam width is denoted by d.

To derive the angular radiation pattern of a rectangular or array element, referring to Figure 3.25 and starting again from the Rayleigh

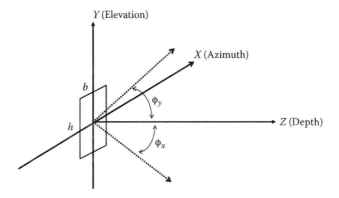

Figure 3.25 Linear array element geometry in 3D.

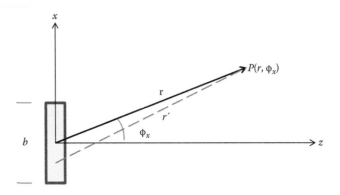

Figure 3.26 Linear array geometry element in 2D.

integral, considering only a 2D case shown in Figure 3.26 for the sake of simplicity and removing the time-dependent term, the pressure at a point (r, φ_x) is given by

$$p(r, \varphi_x) = \frac{jk\rho c}{2\pi} \int_{-b/2}^{b/2} \frac{u(x)e^{-jkr'}}{r'} dx \qquad (3.32)$$

By invoking the law of cosine,

$$r' = \sqrt{r^2 + x^2 + 2rx\sin\varphi_x} \qquad (3.33)$$

Again, making the approximation $\sqrt{1+\delta} \approx 1 + \frac{1}{2}\delta$ if $\delta \sim 0$. Equation (3.33) becomes

$$r' \sim r + x\sin\varphi_x + \frac{x^2}{2r}$$

for $r \gg 6$. Substituting this relation into Equation (3.32), make the approximation $r' \approx r$ in the denominator, but in the exponent $r' \approx r + x\sin\varphi_x$, where only the second-order term is ignored because k is a large number and a small change in r' can cause a large change in the phase term (kr'). Let $\sin \varphi_x$ be represented by δ; Equation (3.32) is reduced to

$$p(r, \delta) = \frac{jk\rho c}{2\pi} \frac{e^{-jkr}}{r} \int_{-b/2}^{b/2} u(x)e^{-jkx\delta} dx \qquad (3.34)$$

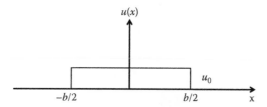

Figure 3.27 Uniform medium-velocity excitation of an array element.

If $u(x)$ on a rectangular aperture is uniformly distributed, i.e., $u(x) = u_0$, as shown in Figure 3.27, it can be easily shown that the angular radiation pattern is a sinc function:

$$H_r(\varphi_x) = H_r(\varphi_x = 0) \frac{\sin\left(kb\dfrac{\sin\varphi_x}{2}\right)}{kb\dfrac{\sin\varphi_x}{2}} \qquad (3.35)$$

which is plotted along with the axial intensity distribution in Figure 3.28 for a 5 MHz rectangular array element of 360 μm wide and 5.1 mm high irradiating into water.

For a rectangular element that is the basic unit of an array with dimension b in the x-direction and h in the y-direction, shown in Figure 3.25, the 3D directivity function is given by

$$H(\varphi_x, \varphi_y) = H(\varphi_x = 0, \varphi_y = 0)\frac{\sin[(kb\sin\varphi_x)/2]}{(kb\sin\varphi_x)/2} \cdot \frac{\sin[(kh\sin\varphi_y)/2]}{(kh\sin\varphi_y)/2} \qquad (3.36)$$

where φ_x and φ_y are angles in the x-z and y-z planes, respectively. The directions of x and y are frequently referred to as the elevational and azimuthal directions in the literature. The ratio $(\sin x)/x$ is the sinc function, which is zero when $x = n\pi$, where n is an integer. Therefore, the first zeros for $H(\varphi_x, \varphi_y)$ are at

$$\varphi_x = \sin^{-1}\frac{\lambda}{b}, \varphi_y = \sin^{-1}\frac{\lambda}{h} \qquad (3.37)$$

For rectangular elements the ratio of the magnitude of the main lobe to that of the first side lobe is –13 dB. The far-field and near-field transition points on the x-z plane and y-z plane occur at $b^2/4\lambda$ and $h^2/4\lambda$, respectively.

The integral in Equation (3.34) actually is the Fourier transform of $u(x)$, defined as the aperture function of the irradiating surface. This observation has a very important ramification, which means that a smoother aperture function suppresses side lobe levels (SSLs). This is evident by examining the SSLs of a circular and a rectangular aperture, which are,

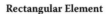

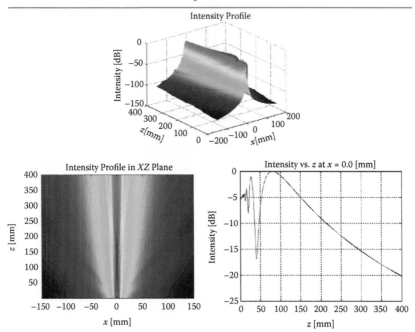

Figure 3.28 Angular and axial intensity distribution of a rectangular array element.

respectively, –17.5 and –13.4 dB down from the main lobe. Moreover if $u(x)$ is Gaussian distributed, the angular radiation pattern of an aperture $H(\delta)$ will also be Gaussian since the Fourier transform of a Gaussian function is also Gaussian. It is therefore possible to suppress SLL by modifying the aperture morphology or applying amplitude weighting to the input electrical signal termed, respectively, aperture and amplitude apodization (Steinberg, 1976; Cobbold, 2007).

The angular radiation pattern $H(\varphi_x)$ depends also on the boundary condition, i.e., how the aperture is supported. $H_r(\varphi_x)$ in Equation (3.35) is for a rigid baffle, which means that the medium surrounding the rectangular aperture is hard and the boundary condition must satisfy that displacement $W(x) = 0$ for $x > (1/2)b$ and $x < -(1/2)b$. $H(\varphi_x)$ should be modified for a soft baffle, the boundary condition of which is pressure $p(x) = 0$ for $x > (1/2)b$ and $x < -(1/2)b$ (Selfridge, 1980), and is given by

$$H_r(\varphi_x) = H_r(\varphi_x = 0)\frac{\sin\left(kb\dfrac{\sin\varphi_x}{2}\right)}{kb\dfrac{\sin\varphi_x}{2}}\cos\varphi_x$$

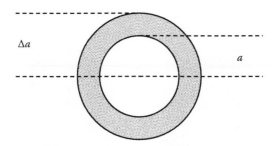

Figure 3.29 A small ring-shaped radiator.

The radiation pattern of a rectangular aperture in a soft baffle is narrower than that in a rigid baffle.

The angular radiation for a ring with Δa much smaller than the wavelength in the loading medium shown in Figure 3.29 is found to be a Bessel function of the first kind of order 0.

$$H_{ring}(\varphi) = H_{ring}(\varphi = 0)J_0(ka\sin\varphi)$$

where the symbols are similar to those shown in Figure 3.20(a). $H_{ring}(\varphi)$ has a narrower beam width, but much higher SSL, in addition to the loss of sensitivity in comparison to a circular aperture because of a smaller aperture area (Cobbold, 2007).

3.5.2 Pulsed ultrasonic field

The above discussion pertains only to continuous-wave propagation. Most applications of ultrasound in medicine, however, involve pulsed ultrasound. From the Fourier transform of the pulse and utilizing the principle of superposition, the field characteristics of a transducer transmitting pulses can be readily calculated. When a transducer is pulsed, the radiation pattern and the field characteristics all become much smoother. Figure 3.30 shows the radiation pattern of a 5 MHz, 1 cm diameter circular piston excited by a one-cycle pulse.

3.5.3 Visualization and mapping of the ultrasonic field

A Schlieren system is an optical device that has been used frequently to visualize the ultrasonic field (Zinskin and Lewin, 1993). As illustrated in Figure 3.31(a), this method depends on the diffraction of a parallel beam of light when it traverses through a medium in which there is a refractive index gradient normal to the light beam. An ultrasonic beam produces such a gradient because the propagation of an ultrasonic wave is

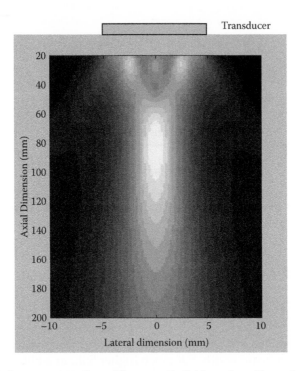

Figure 3.30 A ≈ representation of the acoustic field produced by a circular piston transducer of 1 cm diameter at 5 MHz.

associated with changes in the density of the medium. If the primary nondiffracted light beam is blocked, the diffracted light, which contains an image of the ultrasound beam can be observed directly on a screen, photographed, or captured by a CCD camera and displayed on a monitor. Figure 3.31(b) is a Schlieren image in the near field of a broken 10 MHz transducer of 1 cm diameter obtained by a Schlieren system (Hanafy and Zanelli, 1991). The beam cannot be properly focused to the axial direction.

Although a qualitative interpretation of the Schlieren image is fairly straightforward, a quantitative analysis of the optical image is difficult (Schneider and Shung, 1996). Alternatively a more time-consuming but well-established method where a nondirectional microprobe or hydrophone is used to scan the field may be employed (Zinskin and Lewin, 1993). In addition to nondirectional, the probe should possess nonselective frequency characteristics or a very broad frequency bandwidth. It should be small in size to avoid the establishment of standing waves and minimize the effect of acoustic field averaging over the transducer face. However, in practice, it is almost impossible to satisfy all these requirements. There are different types of hydrophones commercially available,

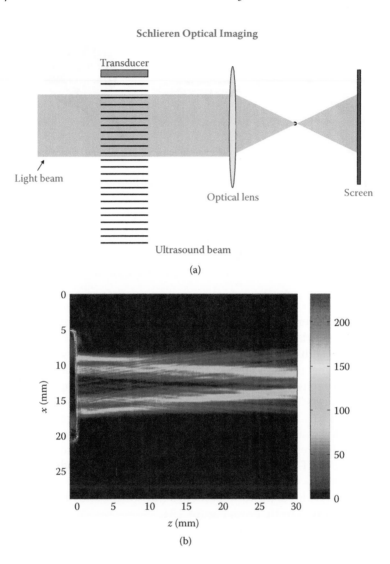

Figure 3.31 (a) The Schlieren optical system for mapping ultrasonic beam characteristics. (b) A Schlieren image of a 10 MHz piston transducer of 1 cm diameter. The transducer is on the left of the image. The diffraction pattern near the transducer is clearly seen. The bar on the right indicates the acoustic intensity.

including the needle type, where the piezoelectric element is housed in a hypodermic needle of less than 1 mm diameter, and the PVDF membrane type, where only the center of a tightly stretched membrane is poled and piezoelectrically active. The diameter of the poled spot for a membrane hydrophone can be made as small as 0.2 mm. A small target such as a

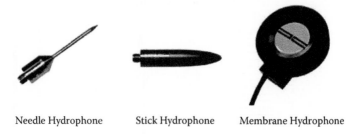

Needle Hydrophone   Stick Hydrophone   Membrane Hydrophone

Figure 3.32 A photo of several hydrophones. (Courtesy of Onda Corp.)

small sphere or wire has also often been used to map the field. A few such hydrophones are shown in Figure 3.32.

3.5.4 Axial and lateral resolutions

The axial and lateral resolutions of a transducer are determined, respectively, by the emitted pulse duration and the beam width of the transducer (−3 dB beam width or −6 dB beam width) because whether the echoes from two targets either in the axial or in the lateral direction can be separated or resolved is directly related to these parameters. This is graphically illustrated in Figure 3.33(a), where it can be seen that the echoes from two targets can be clearly resolved if they are far apart. As the targets are moved closer and closer, as shown in Figure 3.33(b) to (d), they become more and more difficult to resolve. Figure 3.33(d) shows what happens when the two targets coincide. The distance in this figure represents either the axial or lateral distance.

The beam width at the focal point of a transducer, d, is linearly proportional to the wavelength. From Figure 3.24,

$$\sin\varphi = 0.61(\lambda/a) = \frac{\frac{d}{2}}{z_0}$$

Rearranging the equation,

$$d = 2.44(z_0/2a)\lambda = 2.44f_\#\lambda \tag{3.38}$$

where $f_\#$ is the f number defined as the ratio of focal distance to aperture dimension, in this case diameter ($z_0/2a$). For a circular transducer of diameter $2a$ and a focal distance of $4a$, the transducer has an $f_\#$ of 2.

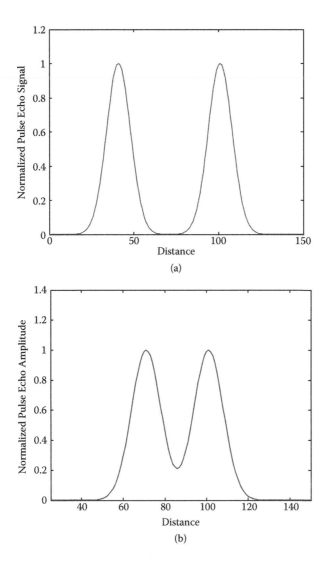

Figure 3.33 The spatial resolutions of an ultrasonic transducer in the axial and lateral directions are determined by the pulse duration and beam width: (a) full width with main lobe separation, (b) half-main lobe width separation, (c) less than half-main lobe width separation, and (d) full width half maximum.

For a rectangular array element, beam widths on the *x-z* plane and *y-z* plane are

$$d_x = 2f_{\#x}\lambda \quad \text{and} \quad d_y = 2f_{\#y}\lambda$$

where $f_{\#x} = z_{0x}/b$ and $f_{\#y} = z_{0y}/h$ are the $f_{\#}$ values on the *x-z* plane and *y-z* plane, respectively.

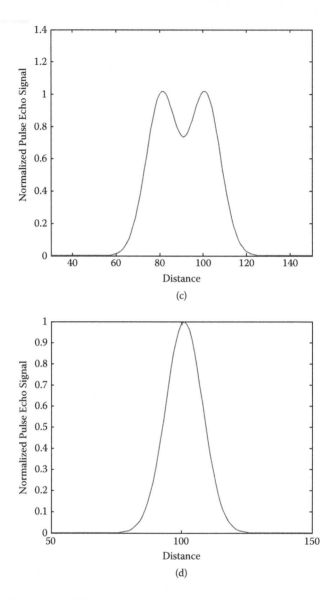

Figure 3.33 *(Continued)* The spatial resolutions of an ultrasonic transducer in the axial and lateral directions are determined by the pulse duration and beam width: (a) full width with main lobe separation, (b) half-main lobe width separation, (c) less than half-main lobe width separation, and (d) full width half maximum.

The depth of focus D_f, that is, within this region the intensity of the beam within -3 dB of the maximal intensity at the focus for a circular aperture and a rectangular aperture, is found to be linearly related to the wavelength (Kino, 1987; McKeighen, 1998).

$$D_{fc} = 7.2 f_\#^2 \lambda \text{ and } D_{fr} = 7.1 f_\#^2 \lambda \qquad (3.39)$$

The depth of field can be defined alternatively as the region between axial distances where the beam widths become $\sqrt{2}d$.

From these relationships, it is clear that an increase in frequency that decreases wavelength improves both lateral and axial resolutions by reducing the beam width and the pulse duration if the number of cycles in a pulse is fixed. Unfortunately, these improvements are achieved at a cost of a shorter depth of focus.

The axial and lateral resolution of a transducer can be improved from an increase in the bandwidth with backing or matching and focusing. The spectrum of an ultrasonic pulse varies as it penetrates into tissue because the attenuation of the tissues is frequency dependent. It is known that the center frequency and bandwidth of an ultrasonic pulse decrease as the ultrasound pulse penetrates deeper. In other words, the axial resolution of the beam worsens as the beam penetrates deeper into the tissue. In commercial scanners, pulse shape and duration are maintained by time gain compensation and some form of signal processing.

3.5.5 Focusing

Better lateral resolution at a certain axial distance can be achieved by acoustic focusing. However, an improvement in the lateral resolution or focusing at a certain range is always accompanied by a loss of resolution in the region beyond the focal zone, as illustrated in Figure 3.34(a).

The general principles of focusing are identical to those in optics. The two most often used schemes, a lens and a spherical or bowl-type transducer, are illustrated in Figure 3.34(a), where z_f and D_f are, respectively, focal distance and depth of focus, and (b). The acoustic lens shown in Figure 3.34(a) is a convex lens, which means that the sound velocity in the lens material is less than the medium into which the beam is launched. The convex lens is preferred in biomedical ultrasonic imaging in that it conforms better to the shape of the body curvature. This is illustrated in Figure 3.35. Some of the lens materials frequently used in medical applications can be found in Table 3.4. The most important requirements are that it should have an acoustic impedance similar to the last matching layer and be slightly attenuative to absorb reverberations

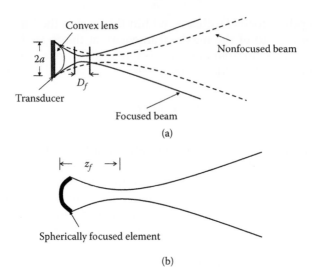

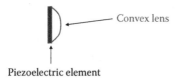

Figure 3.34 Two modes of focusing that have been used to focus ultrasonic beams: (a) focusing with a lens and (b) self-focusing.

of signals inside the lens. As illustrated in Figure 3.36, the focal length z_f of a lens is given by

$$z_f = \frac{R_c}{1-1/n} \tag{3.40}$$

where R_c is the radius of curvature and $n = c_1/c_2$, c_1 is the velocity in the lens and c_2 is being that in the medium. A popular material for convex

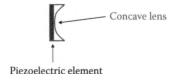

Figure 3.35 Convex and concave lenses.

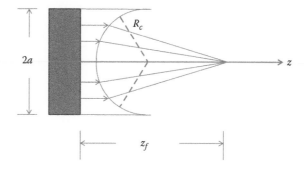

Figure 3.36 Focusing geometry.

lens is RTV silicon rubber, which has a velocity of 1010 m/s, acoustic impedance of 1.5 MRayl, and attenuation of 7 dB/cm-MHz. For a silicon rubber lens in water and a focal distance of 4 cm, R_c can be readily calculated to be 2.12 cm from Equation (3.40). Concave lenses made of polyurethane or polystyrene have also been used. For concave transducers a suitable filler material is needed to make the transducer face flat. Polyurethane has been shown to fit this need. The focal region formed by an acoustic lens is usually ellipsoidal. Its dimension depends on the relationship between wavelength and the diameter of the lens. In general, the bigger the diameter, the smaller the focal point. Ultrasonic imaging is diffraction limited because the beam cannot be properly focused in the region close to the transducer and beyond the near-field and far-field transition point. For a circular piston transducer of radius a, $z_0 = a^2/\lambda$. The $f_\#$ is $a/(2\lambda)$, which is determined by the ratio of radius to wavelength. For a ratio of radius to wavelength $= 10$, $f_\# = 5$. This means that the beam cannot be focused beyond an $f_\#$ of 5. The only way to obtain focusing at a distance greater than this is to either increase the aperture size or decrease the wavelength.

3.5.6 Protection circuits for transducers

Large signals in the order of 100 peak-to-peak volts are needed to drive a transducer. The receiving electronics must be protected from these high voltages (Lockwood et al., 1991; Cobbold, 2007). Figure 3.37(a) shows a protection scheme that is commonly used. R_s, C_s, and L_c represent source output resistance, capacitance, and inductance for a matching network. The load resistance R_l should be much larger than the input resistance of the receiving electronics, R_i, which is in general 50 Ω. When the source is on, both diodes D1 and D2 appear to be shorted. During transmission and reception the circuit behaves like the circuit shown in Figure 3.37(b)

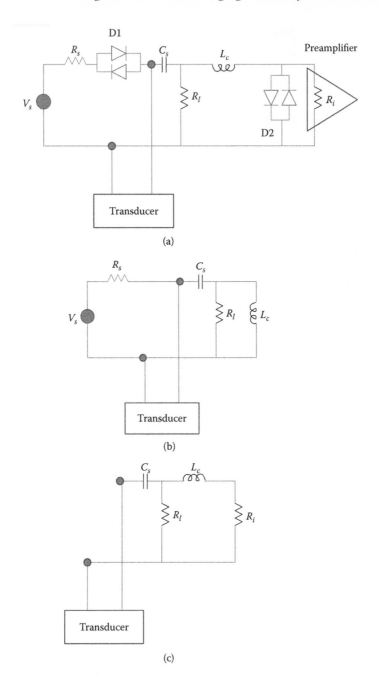

Figure 3.37 (a) A commonly used transducer protection circuit. (b) and (c) Circuit during transmission and reception.

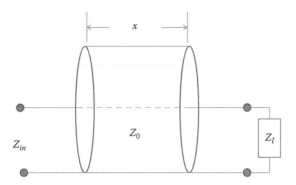

Figure 3.38 An electrical cable terminated by load impedance Z_l.

and (c). At high frequencies (>20 MHz), the cable length may be changed or tuned to match to R_i. The input electrical impedance to a cable shown in Figure 3.38 is given by

$$Z_{in} = Z_0 \frac{Z_l + Z_0 \tanh \gamma x}{Z_0 + Z_l \tanh \gamma x} \tag{3.41}$$

where γ is a complex number $= \alpha + j\beta$, $\alpha =$ attenuation coefficient of the cable, $\beta =$ propagation constant for an electromagnetic wave, and $Z_0 =$ characteristic electrical impedance of the cable. Assuming a lossless cable, Equation (3.41) becomes

$$Z_{in} = Z_0 \frac{Z_l + jZ_0 \tan \beta x}{Z_0 + jZ_l \tan \beta x}$$

At 50 MHz the electromagnetic wavelength is 600 cm, and the cable needs to be considered. If Z_l is zero, when x is $\lambda/4 = 150$ cm in this case, $\beta x = \pi/2$, $\tan\beta_x = \infty$, and $Z_{in} = \infty$. It means that the electrical impedance from the transducer looking into the receiving electronics is ∞ or an open circuit. Another observation is that if $Z_l = Z_0$, $Z_{in} = Z_0$ for all x. If the transducer output impedance is Z_0, the load is matched to the transducer independent of the cable length.

A single-element transducer can be translated or steered mechanically to form an image. Linear translators do not allow movements permitting generation of images at a rate higher than a few frames per second, although there are sector scanning devices that allow steering the transducer within a limited angle at a rate of 30 frames per second. Early real-time ultrasonic imaging devices almost exclusively used this type of transducer, which is called mechanical sector probe. A typical mechanical

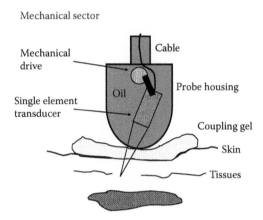

Figure 3.39 Detailed construction of a mechanical sector probe.

sector probe is shown in Figure 3.39. The transducer is housed in a dome bathed in some form of oil to facilitate the transmission of the ultrasonic energy from the transducer to the housing. Mechanical sector probes that suffer from poor near-field image quality because of reverberations between the transducer and the housing and fixed focusing capability have now been largely replaced by linear arrays.

3.6 Arrays

Arrays are transducer assemblies with more than one element. These elements may be rectangular in shape and arranged in a line, called linear array or 1D array, shown in Figure 3.40(a), or square in shape and arranged in rows and columns, called two-dimensional (2D) array, shown in Figure 3.40(b), or ring shaped and arranged concentrically, called annular array, shown in Figure 3.40(c).

A linear switched array (sometimes called a linear sequence or simply a linear array) is operated by applying voltage pulses to groups of elements in succession, as shown in Figure 3.41, where the solid line and the dashed line indicate, respectively, the first and second beams. In this way, the sound beam is moved across the face of the transducer electronically producing a picture similar to that obtained by scanning a single-element transducer manually. The amplitude of the voltage pulses can be uniform or varied across the aperture as shown in the figure by arrows of varying length. As mentioned previously, amplitude apodization or varying the input pulse amplitude across the aperture is sometimes used to suppress side lobes at the expense of worsening the lateral resolution. If the electronic sequencing or scanning is repeated fast enough (30 frames per second), a real-time image can be generated. Linear arrays are usually

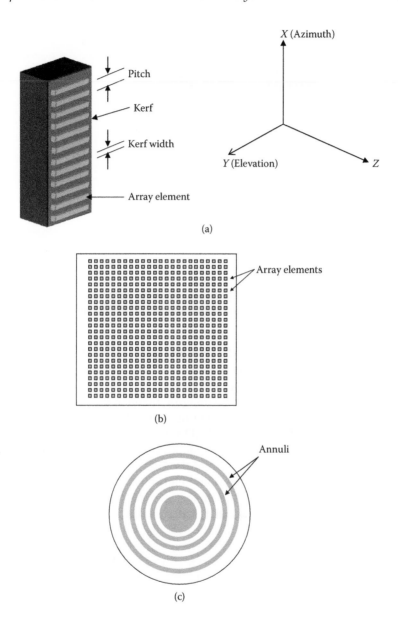

Figure 3.40 (a) A linear array. (b) A 2D array. (c) An annular array.

1 cm wide and 10 to 15 cm long with 128 to 256 elements. Typically 32 or more elements are fired in a group. For the sake of achieving as good a lateral resolution as possible, the irradiating aperture size must be made as large as possible. The aperture size is in turn limited by the requirement of maintaining a large number of scan lines. This point will become

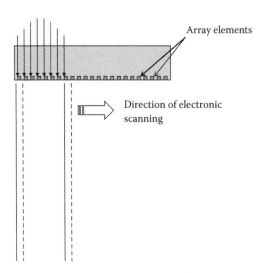

Figure 3.41 An image is formed by a linear array by electronically sweeping the beam. A group of elements are fired simultaneously to form one beam.

clearer in Chapter 4. Figure 3.42 shows the detailed construction of a linear array consisting of a backing material, a layer of piezoelectric material sandwiched between two electrodes, and two matching layers. Here a concave lens is used to focus the imaging plane in the elevational direction or the slice thickness of the imaging plane. This is a problem of crucial importance in 2D imaging with 1D arrays because the slice thickness cannot be controlled throughout the depth of view. The slice thickness is the thinnest only at the focal point of the lens and becomes worse closer to the array or beyond the focal point. Figure 3.43 illustrates how a large slice thickness can cause serious image artifacts, including reduction in contrast. The top panel shows that scatterers outside of the cyst region can cause the echogenicity within the cyst to increase in the field of view where the slice thickness is large. The lower panel shows that although the location of the cyst farther from the transducer is not on the same imaging plane as the cyst closer to the transducer, an ultrasonic image will not be able to tell the difference.

In Figures 3.40(a) and 3.44, the space between two elements is called a kerf and the distance between the centers of two elements is called a pitch. The kerfs may be filled with acoustic isolating material or simply air to minimize acoustic cross talk. The kerfs are often cut into the lens and backing to minimize acoustic cross talk between adjacent elements through the backing, the lens, and matching layers. The size of a pitch in a linear array ranges from $\lambda/2$ to $3\lambda/2$, where λ is the wavelength in the medium into which ultrasound is launched

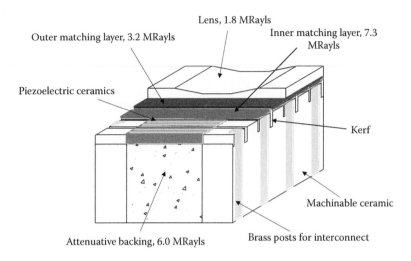

Figure 3.42 Detailed construction of a linear array with two matching layers, a lens, and light backing.

and is not as critical as in a phased array (Steinberg, 1976; Shung and Zipparo, 1996).

The linear phased array, while similar in construction, is quite different in operation. A phased array is smaller (1 cm wide and 1 to 3 cm long) and usually contains fewer elements (96 to 256). Referring to Figure 3.45,

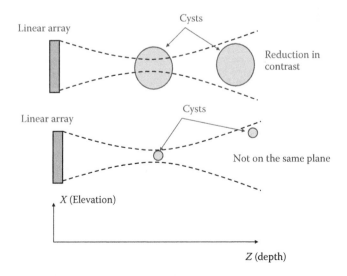

Figure 3.43 Slice thickness causes deleterious artifacts in an image.

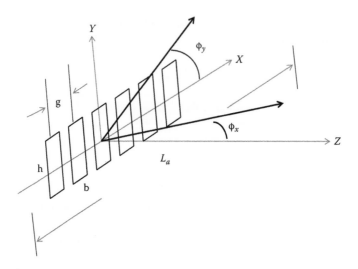

Figure 3.44 Linear array geometry in 3D.

if the difference in path length between the center element and element number n is $\Delta r_n = r - r_n$, at a point $P(r,\varphi_x)$, the time difference is then

$$\Delta t_n = \frac{\Delta r_n}{c} = \frac{x_n \sin \varphi_x}{c} + \frac{x_n^2}{2cr} \tag{3.42}$$

where the first and second terms on the right-hand side of the equation indicate the time differences due to, respectively, steering and

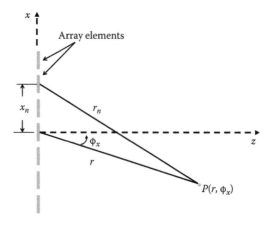

Figure 3.45 A 2D coordinate system depicting the difference in path length between the center element of a linear array and the nth element.

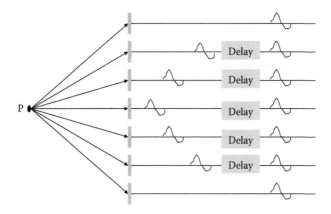

Figure 3.46 The echoes returned from a point scatterer at point P can be made to arrive at the same time by appropriately delaying the echoes detected at the elements of a linear array.

focusing. Therefore, the pulse exciting the center element should be delayed by a time period of Δt_n relative to the pulse exciting the nth element if the ultrasonic pulses are to arrive at point P simultaneously. The ultrasonic beam generated by a phased array can be both focused and steered by properly delaying the signals going to the elements for transmission or arriving at the elements for receiving, as illustrated in Figure 3.46 according to Equation (3.42). To find the radiation pattern in the far field of a linear array of length L_a consisting of N elements, i.e., $z > L_a^2/4\lambda$, a 2D case is assumed here neglecting the elevational or Y dimension, illustrated in Figure 3.47. Assuming first that each array element of the N elements can be represented by a medium-velocity impulse with magnitude u_0, delineated in Figure 3.48, the

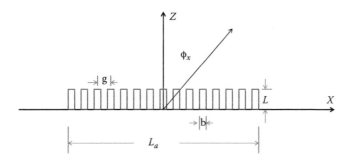

Figure 3.47 Linear array geometry in 2D.

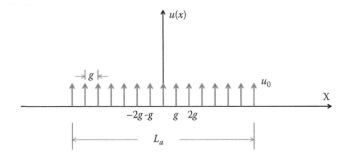

Figure 3.48 Linear array elements are represented by impulses.

mathematical representation of an aperture consisting of an infinite number of impulses is given by

$$u(x) = u_0 \sum_{n=-\infty}^{\infty} \Delta(x \pm ng)$$

where Δ denotes a delta function and n is an interger. The radiation pattern or directivity of such an aperture function, $H(\varphi_x)$, can be found by taking the spatial Fourier transform of $u(x)$ as previously discussed. Assuming $\delta = \sin\varphi_x$,

$$H(\sin\varphi_x) = H(\delta) = u_0 \text{FT} \sum_{n=-\infty}^{\infty} \Delta(x \pm ng) = H(0) \sum_{m=-\infty}^{\infty} \Delta\left(\delta \pm m\frac{\lambda}{g}\right)$$

where $H(0)$ is the directivity at $\delta = 0$. For a series of impulses confined within a length L_a, which is the total length of the array, i.e., a finite aperture, the aperture function $u(x)$ should be modified to

$$u(x) = u_0 \ rect(x) \times \sum_{n=-\infty}^{\infty} \Delta(x \pm ng)$$

where $rect(x)$ represents a rectangular function $= 1$ when $-L_a/2 < x < L_a/2$ and $= 0$ otherwise. The directivity of this aperture function consisting of N impulses confined within a length of L_a is then given by

$$H(\delta) = u_0 \text{FT}[rect(x)]^*\text{FT} \sum_{n=1}^{N} \Delta(x \pm ng) = H(0) sinc\frac{kL_a\delta}{2} * \sum_{m=1}^{N} \Delta\left(\delta \pm m\frac{\lambda}{g}\right)$$

$$(3.43)$$

where * denotes convolution. The result is shown in Figure 3.49, which indicates that at $\delta = \sin\varphi_x = m\lambda/g$, where $m = 1$ to N, there is constructive

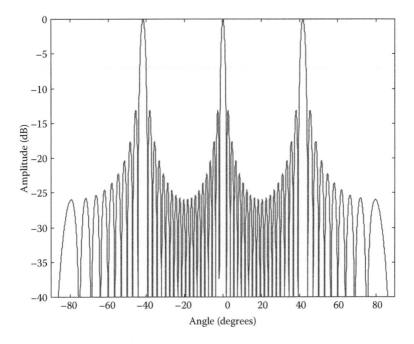

Figure 3.49 Large grating lobes are produced at 40° and −40° by a linear array with an undesirable pitch.

interference, which is called the grating lobe. Grating lobes are very undesirable in imaging because they cause degradation of image contrast and artifacts.

For a linear array consisting of N elements, as shown in Figure 3.47, the aperture function in Equation (3.43) should be replaced by the convolution of the impulses with another rectangular function, $rect'(x) = 1$ when $-b/2 < x < b/2$ and $= 0$ otherwise. Consequently, the radiation pattern $H_a(\varphi_x)$ of a linear array of length L_a and N elements with element width b is given by

$$H_a(\delta) = u_0 \mathrm{FT}[rect(x)] * \mathrm{FT} \sum_{n=1}^{N} \Delta(x \pm ng) * \mathrm{FT}[rect'(x)]$$

$$= H_a(0) \operatorname{sin} c \frac{kL_a\delta}{2} * \sum_{m=1}^{N} \Delta\left(\delta \pm m \frac{\lambda}{g}\right) \times \operatorname{sin} c \frac{kb\delta}{2}$$

Rearranging this equation,

$$H_a(\delta) = \operatorname{sin} c\left(\frac{b\delta}{\lambda}\right) \times \sum_{m=1}^{N} \Delta\left(\delta \pm m \frac{\lambda}{g}\right) * \operatorname{sin} c\left(\frac{L_a\delta}{\lambda}\right) \qquad (3.44)$$

where sinc denotes the sinc function = sinx/x. As discussed, for arrays with regularly spaced elements, high side lobes called grating lobes occur at certain angles because of constructive interference, which is related to the wavelength and the pitch by the following equation:

$$\varphi_{xg} = \sin^{-1}\left(\frac{m\lambda}{g}\right) \qquad (3.45)$$

where m is an integer = ±1, ±2, ... For the grating lobes to occur at angles greater than 90°, g has to be smaller than $\lambda/2$. When this condition is satisfied, the array is said to be fully sampled. Figure 3.50 shows the radiation pattern of a 5 MHz 32-element array with 1.6λ pitch and b = 1.2λ for soft kerf filler material. Here L_a = 51.2λ and the acceptance angle of an array is defined as the angle span between the angles where the envelope drops to zero or $\varphi_{acceptance}$ = 2sin^{-1}(λ/b) = 112.9°. The grating lobes occur at ±38.7°. The first zeros for the main beam occur at φ_x = ±1.1°. The angles where the grating lobes occur clearly from Equation (3.45) are determined by the pitch. The grating lobes move away from the main lobe as the pitch is reduced. Equation (3.44) and Figure 3.50 also show that the magnitude of grating lobe relative to the main lobe is determined by the width of the element, b. The smaller the value for b, the larger the magnitude of grating lobes relative to the main lobe. The width of the main lobe in turn is determined by L_a, the width of the array. The greater the L_a, the smaller the main lobe. There are ways, albeit not perfect, to suppress the grating lobes. These include randomizing the spacings between elements, which

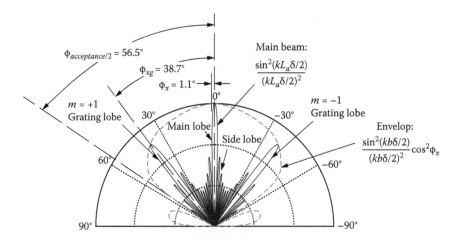

Figure 3.50 Radiation pattern of a 32-element 5 MHz linear array of 1.2λ pitch.

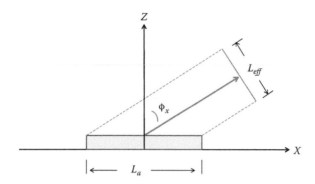

Figure 3.51 For a phased array, as the beam is steered, lateral spatial resolution deteriorates because the effective aperture size decreases.

spread the grating lobe energy in all directions, resulting in a "pedestal" side lobe (Turnbull and Foster, 1992), and subdicing the elements.

There are a few simple design rules for linear arrays and linear phased arrays. For linear arrays, the pitch g should be between 0.75 and 2λ, the ratio of the width of the array element to the thickness of the element (b/L) < 0.6 to avoid spurious lateral resonant modes, $b > \lambda/2$, and the cross talk between adjacent elements < −30 dB. For phased arrays, the pitch g should be smaller than 0.5λ, $b/L < 0.6$, $b \sim \lambda/2$ to ensure a broad beam since the beam is steered, and the cross talk < −35 dB since cross talk can result in an increase in the apparent aperture size. Cross talk for arrays is undesirable because it lengthens ring downtime of the pulse, thus degrading axial resolution. In addition, it causes an increase in effective aperture size. For linear array, it is advantageous in that cross talk in fact sharpens the lateral beam width. It is, however, deleterious for phased array, for which a broader beam is needed for beam steering. Another problem with phased array is that the effective array length decreases as the beam is steered, as shown in Figure 3.51, causing a drop in sensitivity and an increase in lateral beam width. The effective length L_{eff} at a steering angle of φx is $L_{eff} = L_a \sin(90° − \varphi_x) = L_a \cos\varphi_x$.

Cross talk in an array may come from the matching layers, the backing structure, and the lens. As a result, in order to minimize the cross talk, the kerf may be cut through the matching layers into the backing if necessary. In addition, many problems that occur in the fabrication process may cause the performance of an array to deviate from the design. Air pockets may form in the bond lines, matching layers and backing block. Cracks may occur in the piezoelectric layer during dicing. Attaching the wire to the electrodes may cause a certain region of the piezoelectric material to depole. There may be partial bonding or uneven bonding in the bond lines. Because of these problems in array manufacturing, the yield of array fabrication is usually

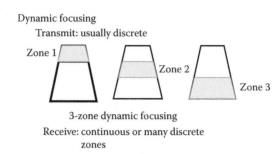

Figure 3.52 Discrete zone dynamic focusing is used for transmission, whereas almost continuous dynamic focusing may be used in reception.

very low at 20%, and as long as the broken elements in an array are less than 4% and are not together, the array is considered commercially acceptable.

Phased arrays allow dynamic focusing and beam steering. Dynamic focusing can be achieved in both transmission and reception. However, multiple transmissions of pulses are needed for dynamic focusing during transmission, slowing down the frame rate. Transmission dynamic focusing is usually done in discrete zones, whereas receiving dynamic focusing can be done in many more zones or almost continuously, as illustrated in Figure 3.52. After all data are acquired, a composite image is formed, taking only the data from the zones where the beam is focused. To maintain the beam width throughout the depth of view, state-of-the-art scanners also use dynamic aperture apodization described earlier, shown in Figure 3.53. The aperture size is varied as a function of time to allow proper focus of the beam at distances D_1, D_2, and D_3. The reduction of

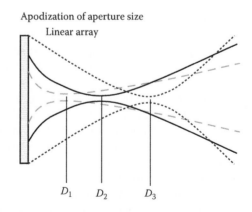

Figure 3.53 Aperture size apodization can be used to maintain the beam width throughout the depth of view.

aperture size is especially crucial in the near field, where the beam cannot be focused for a transducer of a given size.

A photo of a 30 MHz 256-element linear array is shown in Figure 3.54(a). The array is connected to a PCB connector via flexible or flex circuits, which serve three functions: (1) signal connection to each element, (2) array ground connection, and (3) mass termination to the ground plane. The flex circuits are 20–50 μm thick polyimide (trade name Kapton by Dupont) containing copper traces of 5–36 μm thick and 70–125 μm wide. The PCB connector is then connected to a system termination box called ZIF (zero insertion force) connector via cable, as illustrated in Figure 3.54(b).

A variation of the linear array is the curved array shown in Figure 3.55(c) that allows the formation of a pie-shaped image without

A 256-Element 30 MHz Linear Array

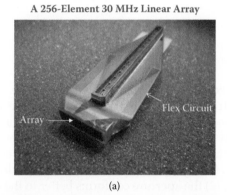

(a)

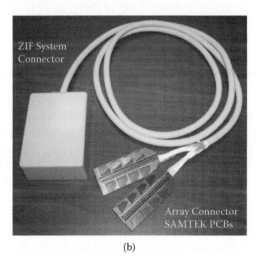

(b)

Figure 3.54 Photos of (a) a linear array and (b) an array connection.

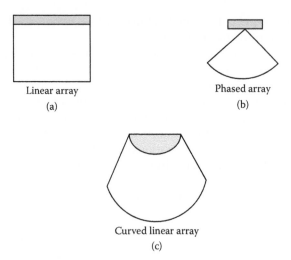

Figure 3.55 The shapes produced by various types of arrays: (a) linear, (b) phased, and (c) curved linear.

resorting to phased array technology, which is more complicated and expensive. In contrast, Figure 3.55(a) and (b) shows the shapes of images obtained by a linear array and a phased array. The advantages of the curved linear array are that (1) the beams are always perpendicular to the aperture, unlike phased arrays, in which the steered beam is affected by the steering angle, losing sensitivity, and lateral resolution as the steering angle is increased; (2) the aperture conforms better to the body surface; (3) it produces an image with a wider field of view; and (4) the pitch does not have to be $\lambda/2$. There are also a couple of disadvantages: (1) larger aperture than phased array and (2) nonuniform scan line density compared to linear array.

Linear arrays can be focused and steered only in one plane, the azimuthal plane. Focusing in the elevation plane perpendicular to the imaging plane, which determines the slice thickness of the imaging plane, is achieved with a lens. This problem may be alleviated by using multidimensional arrays, 1.5D or 2D arrays (Daft et al., 1994; Smith et al., 1995; Shung and Zipparo, 1996). A 1.5D design that is used to provide limited focusing capability in the elevational plane and to reduce slice thickness is shown in Figure 3.56. It is an alternative to 2D arrays, which are still under intensive investigation and are not yet widely commercially available (Smith et al., 1995). In 1.5D arrays, the additional elements in the elevation direction increase the number of electronic channels and complexity in array fabrication. Two concerns associated with 1.5D arrays that do not exist in 1D arrays are grating lobes in the elevational plane as a result of the small number of elements and increased footprint or aperture size.

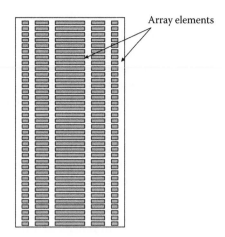

Figure 3.56 A 1.5D array with 5 columns.

Two-dimensional arrays shown in Figure 3.40(b) have been investigated to perform high-speed 3D ultrasonic imaging for cardiac applications (Smith et al., 1995; Greenstein et al., 1997). Current commercial 2D arrays may consist of more than $90 \times 90 = 8100$ elements at 2.5 to 3.5 MHz with fewer than a few hundred elements actually wired. The 2D arrays reported by Greenstein et al. (1997) had $50 \times 50 = 2500$ elements. The square array aperture had a size of 1.5×1.5 cm, with each square element having an area of 250×250 μm. It had one matching layer and a backing with conductive wires embedded in it for electrical connection. Micro-balloon-filled epoxy was used as the kerf filler to reduce cross talk. A unique connection scheme was used to connect the array to the system. The bandwidth was about 50% and cross talk less than −40 dB. The uniformity of responses from individual elements, however, is rather poor.

The 2D array suffers from a severe difficulty in electrical interconnection due to the large number of elements and channels, as well as low signal-to-noise ratio due to electrical impedance mismatching and small element size. Fiber optics and multilayer architecture are possible solutions to the interconnection problem and array stack design. It has been reported that the recently introduced 4D scanner capable of displaying 3D images in real time by Philips incorporates a 2D array of 9212 elements. A novel beamforming scheme in which beamforming is carried out in groups of elements is used to reduce the total number of electronic channels to a manageable level (Savord and Soloman, 2003). An alternative to solving the complexity and cost in electronics and interconnection would be to use sparse array technology that reduces the element and channel count at the price of a poorer signal-to-noise ratio and array performance (Lockwood and Foster, 1996).

The annular arrays shown in Figure 3.40(c) can also achieve biplane focusing. With appropriate externally controllable delay lines or dynamic focusing, focusing throughout the field of view can be attained. A major disadvantage of annular arrays is that mechanical steering has to be used to generate 2D images. In addition, the directivity generated by a ring of radius a is related to $J_0[ka(\sin\varphi_x)]$, which is the Bessel function of the first kind of order 0 (Cobbold, 2007). The main lobe is 25% narrower than a disc of similar radius, but the side lobe level is only –8 dB relative to the main lobe. The areas of all annuli in a typical annular array design are made equal to insure that the beam intensity generated by and the input electrical impedance at each annulus are similar. Another approach utilizes the so-called Fresnel pitch, illustrated in Figure 3.57. The path difference between each ring and the center element is made to equal $2n\pi$ to minimize phase differences of pulses arriving at the focal point, i.e.,

$$k\Delta z_n = k(z_n - z_0) = k\left(\sqrt{r_n^2 + z_0^2} - z_0\right) = 2n\pi$$

This equation can be simplified to

$$\sqrt{r_n^2 + z_0^2} - z_0 = n\lambda$$

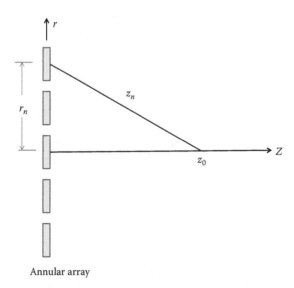

Annular array

Figure 3.57 Cross-sectional view of a Fresnel pitch annular array on the y-z or x-z plane.

Thus,

$$r_n = \sqrt{n\lambda(2z_0 + n\lambda)}$$

It should be noted that Fresnel pitch and equal area cannot be achieved at the same time.

3.6 Characterization of transducer/ array performance

A number of parameters have been used to assess the performance of a transducer/array. Chief among them are insertion loss, cross talk level, pulse-echo test, directivity function, and axial pressure profile. Methods that have been used to measure insertion and cross talk are described below. Others have been discussed in previous sections.

3.6.1 Insertion loss

Insertion loss (IL) is a traditional measurement of transducer sensitivity. Different schemes have been developed for IL measurements (Foster et al., 1991; Ritter et al., 2002). One of these experimental arrangements is shown in Figure 3.58. The reflector, which can be focused or flat, is placed at the focal point of the transducer. To measure the reference signal V_r, the switch is placed at position 2, the open position, and the scope input is set to be 50 Ω. To measure the received echo signal V_e, the switch is placed

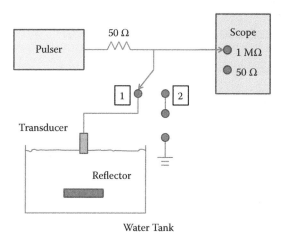

Figure 3.58 Experimental arrangement for measuring insertion loss of a transducer.

at position 1, and the scope input is set to be 1 MΩ. The insertion loss of the transducer expressed in dB can then be calculated from the following equation:

$$IL = 20\log\frac{V_e}{V_r}$$

IL depends upon the aperture size of the transducer and the shape of the reflector, which can be either flat or spherical. Therefore, it is very difficult to compare the values from different laboratories. In the clinical frequency range, for large single-element transducers, IL should be around −5 dB, whereas for linear array and 2D elements it should be around −20 and −40 dB, respectively.

3.6.2 Cross talk

Two cross talk measurements are typically made for array transducers: cross talk levels during transmission and during reception (Smith et al., 1991). Figure 3.59(a) and (b) show, respectively, the experimental arrangements that are used for measuring transmission and reception cross talk levels. In the transmission cross talk measurement, a signal generator with 50 Ω output impedance drives one element at a voltage V_{rt}, and the signal detected at a neighboring element with a scope with either 50 Ω or 1 MΩ input V_{ct} is measured. The transmission cross talk level (CTL_t) is given by

$$CTL_t = 20\log\frac{V_{ct}}{V_{rt}}$$

Scope input at either 50 Ω or 1 MΩ has been used.

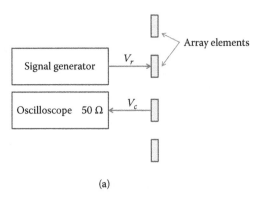

(a)

Figure 3.59 Experimental arrangement for measuring cross talk of a transducer during (a) transmission and (b) reception.

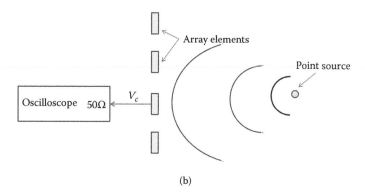

(b)

Figure 3.59 (Continued) Experimental arrangement for measuring cross talk of a transducer during (a) transmission and (b) reception.

In the reception cross talk measurement, a point source, i.e., a transducer with a small aperture, is placed in the far field of the array and the signal at an element is measured with a scope with either 50 Ω or 1 MΩ input, V_{cr}. Another measurement of the signal at the element is then made with all other elements shorted, V_{rr}. The reception cross talk level (CTL_r) is given by

$$CTL_r = 20\log\frac{V_{cr} - V_{rr}}{V_{rr}}$$

Cross talk measurements may also be performed on elements other than the neighboring elements.

References and Further Reading Materials

ANSI/IEEE. Standard on piezoelectricity, STD 176-1987. New York: IEEE, 1987.

Brown LF. Design considerations for piezoelectric polymer ultrasound transducers. *IEEE Trans Ultrasonics Ferroelect Freq Cont* 2000: 47; 1377–1396.

Cady WG. *Piezoelectricity*. New York: Dover, 1964.

Cubbold RSC. *Foundations of biomedical ultrasound*. Oxford, UK: Oxford University Press.

Daft CMW, Wildes DG, Thomas LJ, and Smith LS. A 1.5 D transducer for medical ultrasound. *IEEE Ultrasonics Symp Proc* 1994; 1491–1495.

Desilets CS, Fraser JD, and Kino GS. The design of efficient broad-band piezoelectric transducers. *IEEE Trans Sonics Ultrasonics* 1978; 25: 115–125.

Foster FS, Ryan LK, and Turnbull DH. Characterization of lead zirconate titanate ceramics for use in miniature high-frequency (20-80 MHz) transducers. *IEEE Trans Ultrasonics Ferroelect Freq Cont* 1991; 38(5):446–53.

Goldberg RL and Smith SW. Transducers. In Bronzino J (ed.), *The biomedical engineering handbook*. Boca Raton, FL: CRC Press, 1994, pp. 1077–1092.

Greenstein M, Lum P, Yoshida H, and Seyed-Bolorforosh MS. A 2.5 MHz array with Z-axis electrically conductive backing. *IEEE Trans Ultrasonics Ferroelect Freq Cont* 1997: 44; 970–982.

Gururaja TR, Schulze WA, Cross LE, Newnham RE, Auld BA, and Wang YJ. Piezoelectric composite materials for ultrasonic transducer applications. Part I. Resonant modes of vibration of PZT rod-polymer composites. *IEEE Trans Sonics Ultrasonics* 1985: 32; 481–498.

Hanafy A and Zanelli CI. Quantitative real-time pulsed Schlieren imaging of ultrasonic waves. *IEEE Ultrasonics Symp Proc* 1991: 1223–1227.

Kino GS. *Acoustic waves*. Englewood Cliffs, NJ: Prentice-Hall, 1987.

Kinsler LE, Frey AR, Coppens AB, and Sanders JV. *Fundamentals of acoustics*. 4th ed. New York: John Wiley, 2000.

Krimholtz R, Leedom D, and Matthaei G. New equivalent circuits for elementary piezoelectric transducers. *Electronics Lett* 1970; 6: 398–399.

Lockwood GR and Foster FS. Optimizing the radiation pattern of sparse periodic linear arrays. *IEEE Trans Ultrasonics Ferroelect Freq Cont* 1996: 43; 7–14.

Lockwood GR, Hunt JW, and Foster FS. Design of protection circuitry for high frequency ultrasound systems. *IEEE Trans Ultrasonics Ferroelect Freq Cont* 1991; 38: 48–55.

McKeighen RE. Design guidelines for medical ultrasonic arrays. *SPIE Proc Ultrasonic Transducer Engineering* 1998; 3341: 2–18.

Newnham RE, Skinner DP, and Cross LE. Connectivity and piezoelectric-pyroelectric composites. *Mater Res Bull* 1978; 13: 525–536.

Ristic VM. *Principles of acoustic devices*. New York: John Wiley, 1983.

Ritter TA, Shrout TR, Tutwiler R, and Shung KK. A 30 MHz composite array for medical imaging applications. *IEEE Trans Ultrasonics Ferroelect Freq Cont* 2002; 49:217–230.

Safari A and Akdogan EK. *Piezoelectric and acoustic materials for transducer applications*. New York: Springer, 2008.

Savord B and Soloman R. Fully sampled matrix transducers for real-time 3D ultrasonic imaging. *IEEE Ultrasonics Symp Proc* 2003; 945–953.

Sayers CM and Tait CE. Ultrasonic properties of transducer backings. *Ultrasonics* 1984: 22; 57–63.

Schneider B and Shung KK. Quantitative analysis of pulsed ultrasonic beam patterns using a Schlieren system. *IEEE Trans Ultrasonics Ferroelect Freq Cont* 1996; 43: 1181–1186.

Selfridge AR. Approximate material properties in isotropic materials. *IEEE Trans Sonic Ultrasonics* 1985: 32; 381–394.

Selfridge AR, Kino GS, and Khuri-Yakub BT. A theory for the radiation pattern of a rectangular narrow-strip acoustic transducer. *J Appl Phys* 1980: 37; 35–36.

Shrout TR and Fielding J Jr. Relaxor ferroelectric materials. *IEEE Ultrasonics Symp Proc* 1990; 711–720.

Shung KK and Zipparo M. Ultrasonic transducers and arrays. *IEEE Eng Med Biol Mag* 1996; 15: 20–30.

Smith SW, Davidson RE, and Emery CD. Update on 2-D array transducers for medical ultrasound. *IEEE Ultrasonics Symp Proc* 1995; 1273–1278.

Smith SW, Pavy HG, and von Ramm OT. High speed ultrasound volumetric imaging system. Part I. Transducer design and beam steering. *IEEE Trans Ultrasonics Ferroelect Freq Cont* 1991; 38: 100–108.

Smith WA. The role of piezocomposites in ultrasonic transducers. *IEEE Ultrasonics Symp Proc* 1989; 755–766.

Steinberg BD. *Principles of aperture and array system design.* New York: John Wiley, 1976.

Thiagarajan S, Jayawyrdena I, and Martin RW. Design of 20 MHz wideband piezo-electric transducers for close-proximity imaging. *Biomed Sci Instrum* 1991; 27: 57–60.

Tian J, Han PD, Huang XL, Pan HX, Carroll JF, and Payne DA. Improved stability for piezoelectric crystal growth in the lead indium niobate–lead magnesium niobate–lead titanate system. *Appl Phys Lett* 2007; 91: 222903.

Turnbull DH and Foster FS. Simulation of B-scan images from two-dimensional arrays. *Ultrasonics Imag* 1992; 14: 323–331.

Zinskin MC and Lewin PA. *Ultrasonic exposimetry.* Boca Raton, FL: CRC Press, 1993.

Zipparo MJ, Shung KK, and Shrout TR. Piezoelectric properties of fine grain PZT materials. *IEEE Trans Ultrasonics Ferroelect Freq Cont* 1997; 44: 1038–1048.

chapter four

Gray-scale ultrasonic imaging

The transducers/arrays described in Chapter 3 are used to generate and receive ultrasound signals required to form an image. In this chapter other crucial components of an imaging system that generates, processes, and displays the ultrasound signal in an image are discussed. Typically the image is displayed in gray scale. It can also be represented by such formats as rainbow or heated object scale, depending on the preference of the manufacturer and the clinical need. It must be stressed that these images yield mostly information about the anatomy of the object being imaged. There are various modes of ultrasound imaging that have been used over the years. Today, most of the ultrasonic imaging systems are digital in nature. However, for the sake of a better understanding of the principles and architecture involved, a discussion of these instruments in the analog form is more desirable.

4.1 A- (amplitude) mode and B- (brightness) mode imaging

A-mode is the simplest and earliest mode of ultrasonic imaging. A block diagram for A-mode instruments is shown in Figure 4.1. A signal generator that produces high-amplitude short pulses or a pulser is used to excite a single-element transducer. Two types of pulses may be used: spike and multicycle, illustrated in Figure 4.2. A spike yields wider bandwidth, whereas multicycle bursts provide more energy and allow tuning capability. The returned echoes from the tissues are detected by the same transducer, amplified, and processed for display. The pulses are repeatedly transmitted typically at a rate of a few kHz, which is called pulse repetition frequency (PRF). PRF determines the depth of penetration of the pulse. In order to avoid range ambiguity, all echoes from targets of interest must be received before the next pulse is transmitted. Otherwise, uncertainty of the actual distance between the echo and source may arise. A coupling medium in the form of an aqueous gel or oil is used to couple the transducer to the body because of the mismatch in acoustic impedance between air and the transducer and between air and the body. Without the gel very little energy can be transmitted into the body. The echoes returned from various structures due to large interfaces between organs or small anatomical structures

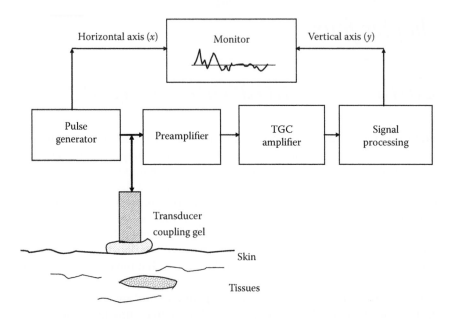

Figure 4.1 Block diagram of an A-mode scanner.

in the organ, such as cells, small blood vessels, ducts, etc. (Shung and Thieme, 1993), are first amplified by a preamplifier. The preamplifier that provides the initial state of signal amplification with a gain of a few dB is an amplifier with high-input electrical impedance and low noise. A second-stage amplification is provided by the time-gain-compensation (TGC) amplifier that may have a gain greater than 40 dB. TGC is needed because ultrasound energy is attenuated by tissues as it penetrates deeper into the body. TGC is usually achieved by a variable

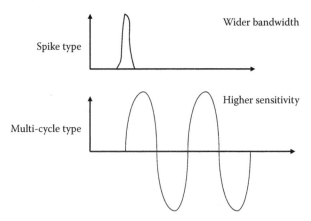

Figure 4.2 Two types of pulses that are used to excite the transducers.

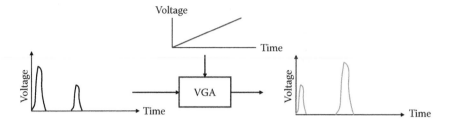

Figure 4.3 Time-gain-compensation can be achieved with a variable gain amplifier.

gain amplifier whose gain is proportional to time so that deeper echoes receive more amplification, as illustrated in Figure 4.3. In this case, the gain is linearly related to time. Energy loss is affected not only by tissue attenuation that is exponentially related to the depth of penetration as previously discussed, but also by beam diffraction. Therefore, it is quite difficult to accurately compensate for the energy loss. A variety of TGC curves, shown in Figure 4.4, have been used and are usually available in an ultrasonic scanner for the operator to select. The amplified signal is then demodulated, involving envelope detection and filtering, and logarithmically compressed. Logarithmic compression, which can be done with a logarithmic amplifier, is needed because the dynamic range of the received echoes, which is defined as the ratio of the largest echo to the smallest echo above noise level detectable by the transducer, is very large, in the order of 100 to 120 dB. Typical display units can only display signals with a dynamic range up to 40 dB at best. The horizontal axis of the display unit is synchronized or triggered by pulses generated by the pulser, whereas the vertical axis or vertical deflection of the electron beam is driven by the output of the signal processing unit, which is the demodulated and log-compressed echo amplitude, or simply the video signal.

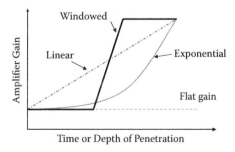

Figure 4.4 Time-gain-compensation curves frequently used in ultrasonic imaging.

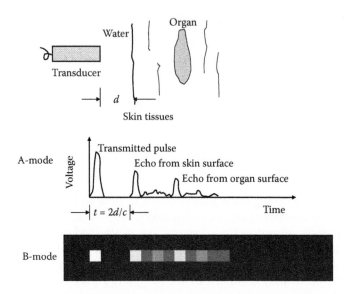

Figure 4.5 A-mode display of returned echoes as a function of time of flight for the arrangement shown on the top of the figure that depicts a transducer sending out a short pulse into the human body and receiving the returned echoes. B-mode display of A-mode data where the echo amplitude in each pixel is represented by gray level. Brighter pixels represent echoes with higher amplitude. Each square denotes a pixel of the display.

The type of information obtained by an A-mode instrument is called an A-line. Figure 4.5 shows an A-line for an arrangement shown on the top of the figure, in which a transducer emits a pulse and the returned echoes from the skin surface and tissue components beneath the skin are received by the same transducer. This information can be displayed in an alternative format, B-mode display, in which the echo amplitude is used to modulate the intensity of the electronic beam of the display unit. Therefore, the echo amplitude is represented by the brightness or gray level of the display. In the bottom of Figure 4.5, a B-mode display of the A-line is shown. Each square in the B-mode display depicts a pixel of the monitor where the brightness is proportional to echo amplitude. It is not necessary to display the echo information in this manner. The echo amplitude or video signal versus gray level mapping can be made adjustable, as illustrated in Figure 4.6, depending upon the clinical application. For example, windowed gray-scale mapping may be used to enhance the image contrast of tissues in regions where there are no strong reflectors or strong echoes that need to be suppressed. This is an option available in commercial scanners. An A-line or single line of the B-mode display yields information about the position of the echo given by $d = ct/2$, where d is the distance from the transducer to the target, t is the time of flight or

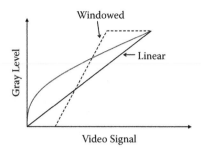

Figure 4.6 Various forms of gray-scale to echo amplitude mapping.

the time needed for the pulse to travel from the transducer to the target and return to the transducer, and c is the sound velocity in the tissues, which is assumed to be a constant of 1540 m/s in commercial scanners, and information about the acoustic properties of the tissues, e.g., size and acoustic impedance. Sound velocity can be assumed to be a constant because sound velocity in tissues does not vary significantly, typically less than 5%, as previously discussed. This assumption may sometimes cause errors in distance, area, or volume measurements and image distortion.

A majority of commercial scanners on the market today are 2D B-mode scanners in which the beam position is also monitored. Figure 4.7 shows a static B-scanner where the position of the transducer in the x-y plane is encoded. The positional information of the beam plus the video signal representing echoes returned from the z-direction are converted into a format that is compatible with a display monitor in a device, called a scan converter, and almost invariably digital today. If the transducer is scanned in the x-direction, then the image formed represents an image of structures in the x-z plane. Images can also be formed by superposition of multiple images after translating and rotating the transducer at a fixed x position within a sector angle, as illustrated in Figure 4.8. This

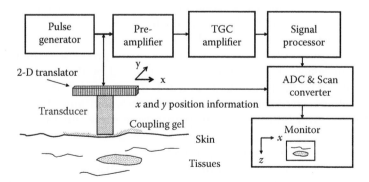

Figure 4.7 Block diagram of a static B-mode scanner.

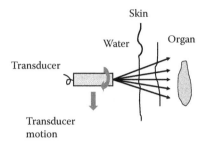

Figure 4.8 Compound scan is performed by combining two different modes of motion of the transducer in forming one image. In this case, the motions are linear translation and rocking of the transducer within a sector angle.

is called compound B-scan. The advantages of doing so are to make the image look smoother or suppress the speckle pattern, which will be discussed later, and to average out the specular echoes due to flat interfaces. The disadvantage is that it slows down the image acquisition rate. Several manufacturers have now included this mode of imaging in their systems, albeit carried out with arrays. The improvement in image quality is quite evident. Static B-scanners are no longer used today because of the poor image quality due to the lack of dynamic focusing and low image acquisition rate, except for high-frequency (20 MHz to 1 GHz) acoustic microscopic applications. Modern B-mode scanners can acquire images faster than 30 frames per second to allow monitoring of organ motion.

Depending upon the mechanisms used to drive a transducer, the real-time scanners are classified into mechanical sector and electronic array scanners. Since electronic array systems generally produce images of better quality, modern ultrasonic scanners are almost exclusively array-based systems. Figure 4.9(a) to (c) shows, respectively, a photograph of a modern ultrasonic scanner, an image of a breast cyst produced by a linear curved array, and an image of the heart produced by a linear phased array in which the color indicates blood flow. Figure 4.9(c) is a color Doppler flow image, which will be discussed in Chapter 6.

The block diagram of an earlier analog B-mode imaging system is shown in Figure 4.10. A pulser is switched on to a group of elements with or without delays. The returned echoes detected by the array elements are processed by the front-end analog beamformer, consisting of a matrix of delay lines, transmit/receive (T/R) switches, and amplifiers. Several components in a B-mode scanner perform the same functions as those in the A-mode system. These include the time-gain-compensation (TGC) amplifier and signal processing units for signal compression, demodulation, and filtering. Various forms of TGC are available on the console for the operator to choose from. The timing and control signals are all generated by a central unit. The image is displayed on a storage monitor.

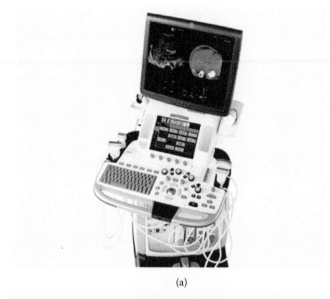

(a)

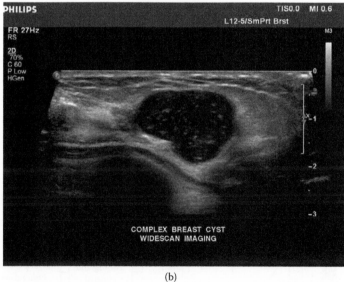

(b)

Figure 4.9 (a) A photo of a modern ultrasonic scanner. (Courtesy of GE Medical Systems.) (b) An image of a lesion in breast obtained by a linear array. (Courtesy of Philips Ultrasound.) (c) A four-chamber view of the heart obtained from the apex of the heart with a phased array. (Courtesy of Philips Ultrasound.)

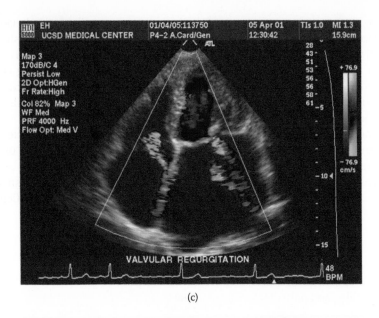

(c)

Figure 4.9 (Continued) (a) A photo of a modern ultrasonic scanner. (Courtesy of GE Medical Systems.) (b) An image of a lesion in breast obtained by a linear array. (Courtesy of Philips Ultrasound.) (c) A four-chamber view of the heart obtained from the apex of the heart with a phased array. (Courtesy of Philips Ultrasound.)

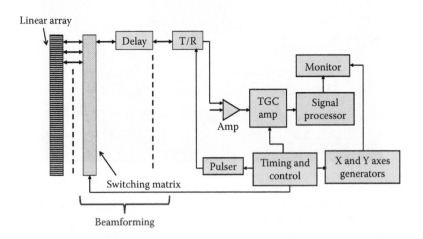

Figure 4.10 Block diagram of an analog ultrasonic imaging system developed in the 1970s.

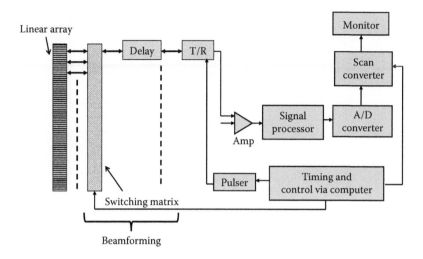

Figure 4.11 Block diagram of a hybrid ultrasonic imaging system where the front end is analog and only the video signal is digitized.

In later systems shown in Figure 4.11 after signal processing, the signal is digitized by an analog-to-digital (A/D) converter. In high-end systems, a digital beamformer, shown in Figure 4.12(a), is used. The A/D conversion following preamplification is accomplished in the beamformer, shown in

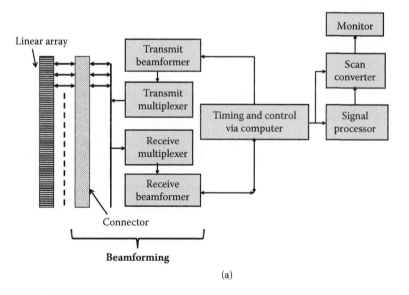

(a)

Figure 4.12 (a) Block diagram of a digital ultrasonic imaging system. (b) Digital receive beamformer from the front end. (*Continued*)

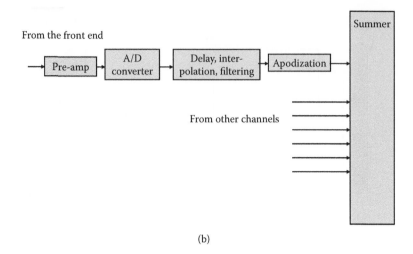

(b)

Figure 4.12 *(Continued)* (a) Block diagram of a digital ultrasonic imaging system.
(b) Digital receive beamformer from the front end.

Figure 4.12(b). This makes the system much more expensive since many
more A/D converters of a higher sampling rate are required. The accuracy of the A/D conversion is determined by the number of bits of the
A/D converter. An 8-bit A/D converter digitizes the signal into $2^8 = 256$
gray level. For better contrast resolution, more bits are needed. High-end
machines display more than 256 gray levels. A/D conversions in a clinical scanner typically have 12-bit accuracy and a 60 MHz sampling rate.
The scan converter is a digital memory device that stores the data that
have been converted from the format in which they were collected into a
format that is displayable by a monitor. The simplest method is to assign
the nearest sample value to the pixel. Inadequate data interpolation causes
a Moiré artifact in sector scanning (Ophir and Maklad, 1979), shown in
Figure 4.13. To remove the Moiré artifact, data interpolation requiring
coordinate transformation of pixels from Cartesian to polar coordinate
is performed. A simple approach is illustrated in Figure 4.14, where the X
values represent the pixels and the solid dots the positions for which echo
data have been acquired. The pixel value is extrapolated from neighboring positions, where echo data are available from the following equation:

$$A_p = \frac{S_1 \times \alpha + S_2 + \beta}{\alpha + \beta}$$

where A_p is the pixel value at point P, and S_1 and S_2 are sampled values or echo data at these positions. There are much more sophisticated
approaches that have been developed.

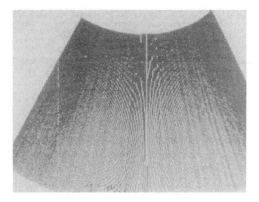

Figure 4.13 Moiré artifact produced by a phased array when the data are under-sampled. (From Ophir and Maklad, *Proceedings of the IEEE* 1979. 67: 654–664.)

Before display, the video data may be processed again via band pass filtering, high-pass filtering, low-pass filtering, gray-scale mapping, etc. Signal processing performed before and after the scan converter is called pre- and post-processing, respectively.

For most of the B-mode scanners, only one ultrasound pulse is being transmitted at any one instant of time. As seen from Figure 4.15, the time needed to form one frame of image, t_f, can be readily calculated from the following equation:

$$t_f = \frac{2DN}{c} \tag{4.1}$$

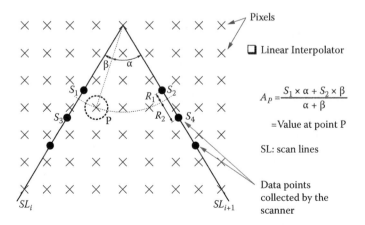

Figure 4.14 Data interpolation in scan conversion.

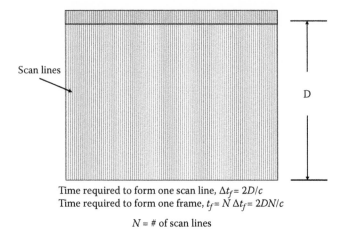

Time required to form one scan line, $\Delta t_f = 2D/c$
Time required to form one frame, $t_f = N\,\Delta t_f = 2DN/c$

$N = \#$ of scan lines

Figure 4.15 Linear array image format.

where D is the depth of penetration determined by the pulse repetition frequency of the pulser, N is the number of scan lines in the image, and c is the sound speed in tissue. Rearranging this equation,

$$FDN = \frac{c}{2} \tag{4.2}$$

where $F = 1/t_f$ is the frame rate. The depth of penetration D is specified by the pulse repetition period of the scanner, which should be long enough to allow all the echoes of interest to be detected. Range ambiguity can result if the pulse repetition period is too short. For instance, range ambiguity can occur, i.e., it is not clear which pulse causes the echo from the object, if the time of flight from an object of interest is longer than the pulse repetition period. Looking at Equation (4.2), it is readily apparent that to change any one of these parameters, F, D, and N, the rest will be affected because sound velocity in tissues is assumed to be a constant. One example is that if the depth of penetration is increased, either the frame rate or the number of scan lines will have to be reduced.

4.1.1 Resolution of B-mode ultrasonic imaging systems

The resolution of a B-mode imaging system in the imaging or azimuthal plane is determined by the duration of the pulse in the depth direction (i.e., in the direction of the beam) and the width of the ultrasonic beam in the lateral direction (i.e., in the direction perpendicular to the beam), as previously discussed. The slice thickness of the imaging plane or the beam width in the elevational plane is fixed and determined by the lens properties.

4.1.2 Beamforming

In real-time imaging with linear arrays, the ultrasonic beam can be dynamically focused and steered by applying appropriate time delays to the transmitted pulses and received echoes utilizing Equation (3.34), as illustrated in Figure 3.45, which shows the top view of several elements of a linear array. Equation (3.34) can be obtained by considering that the difference in the path length between the nth element and the center element is $\Delta r = r_n - r$, where from the cosine law r_n is given by

$$r_n = [r^2 + x_n^2 - 2rx_n \cos(90^0 + \varphi_x)]^{1/2}$$

$$= [r^2 + x_n^2 + 2rx_n \sin(90^0 + \varphi_x)]^{1/2}$$

$$\therefore \Delta r_n = r \left[\frac{(r^2 + x_n^2 + 2rx_n \sin \varphi_x)^{1/2}}{r} - 1 \right]$$

By making the assumption that $r \gg x_n$, that is, the point P is in the far field of the array, and using the approximation $(1 + x)^{1/2} \sim 1 + (1/2)x$ for $x \sim 0$, this equation can be simplified to

$$\therefore \Delta r_n \approx x_n \sin \varphi_x + \frac{x_n^2}{2r}$$

The timing needs to be adjusted to make the transmitted pulse emitted by each element relative to other elements arrive at point P at the same time. The time delay of the transmitted pulse to the center element relative to the nth element is therefore given by Equation (3.34), which is

$$\Delta t_n = \Delta r_n / c \approx \frac{x_n \sin \varphi_x}{c} + \frac{x_n^2}{2cr}$$

where the first and second terms represent, respectively, the time delays needed for achieving beam steering and focusing. The same criteria can be applied to the receiving beam or the echo returned from point P. A delay of Δt_n to the echo received by the center element is needed to make the echo and the echo received by the nth element be summed at the same time, illustrated in Figure 3.45.

This time delay function is one of the functions provided by the beamformer of the ultrasonic imaging system. Other functions of the beamformer are weighting and apodization of the transmitted and received signals. In earlier days, the beamforming was predominantly accomplished with analog devices or by analog beamformers. The problems of these devices are bulky delay lines, incapability of finer delays, electrical impedance mismatch, limited bandwidth, switching transients, and insertion loss. Digital beamformers are used today in most high-end systems. A digital beamformer is primarily a sampling-delay-sum-detection process, as opposed to the delay-sum-detection-sampling process in analog systems. As was discussed, a drawback of the digital beamformers is their cost, which increases with the number of array elements and electronic channel counts. Currently digital beamformers in commercial scanners sample the data at 60 to 80 MHz to 10 to 12 bits.

Mathematically the beamforming function can be summarized by the following equation (Thomenius, 1996):

$$e(t) = \sum_{i=1}^{N} A_{ri} \sum_{j=1}^{N} A_{tj} V\left[t - \Delta t_{ri} - \Delta t_{tj} + \frac{2r(t)}{c}\right] \tag{4.3}$$

where $e(t)$ is the summed echo waveform at the summing amplifier, $V(t)$ is the transmitted waveform, N is the number of array elements, $r(t)$ is the focal distance at a particular time, A_{ri} and A_{tj} are the weighting functions for reception at channel i and transmission at channel j, and Δt_{tj} and Δt_{ri} are, respectively, the time delays applied during transmission and reception to elements j and i. For uniform excitation and receive weighting, $A_{tj} = 1$ and $A_{ri} = 1$. For systems that use fixed transmission focusing, this equation is reduced to

$$e(t) = \sum_{i=1}^{N} V\left[t - \Delta t_{ri} + \frac{2r(t)}{c}\right] \tag{4.4}$$

4.1.3 Speckle

B-mode ultrasonic images exhibit a granular appearance, called speckle pattern, which is caused by the constructive and destructive interferences of the wavelets scattered by the tissue components as they arrive at the transducer surface, as shown in Figure 4.16 (Wagner et al., 1983; Shung and Thieme, 1993). The speckle pattern becomes more obvious at higher frequencies. Figure 4.17 shows an image of a layer of the human vocal cord tissue obtained *in vitro* at 47 MHz. This speckle appearance very much

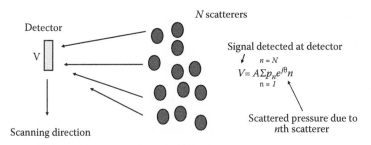

Figure 4.16 The signal detected at a transducer or element is the summation of all scattered echoes generated by the scatterers in the ultrasound beam.

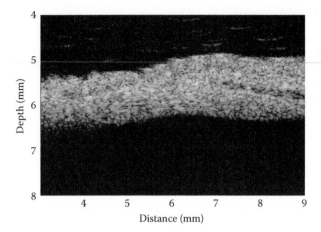

Figure 4.17 An ultrasound image of a human vocal cord tissue at 47 MHz.

resembles the speckle pattern that results from laser scattering by a rough surface. If the incident ultrasound beam is totally coherent like the laser beam, the speckle carries no information about the microstructure of the tissues. Fortunately, ultrasonic scanners use partially coherent incident waves, i.e., pulses. Thus, the speckle patterns exhibited by tissues do contain useful information about the structures of the tissues, which can be used clinically for tissue differentiation.

The resemblance between laser and ultrasound speckles has been extensively analyzed (Wagner et al., 1983). The histogram of the video signals or echo amplitude returned from tissues or the number of occurrences plotted as a function of the amplitude of these echoes V follows a Rician distribution, shown in Figure 4.18, similar to the distribution of the magnitude of a phasor $V = X + jY$ with a uniform phase, as illustrated in Figure 4.19(a) and (b). The symbol σ^2 denotes the variance of the real component X or imaginary component Y. This means that the signal contains random and ordered components. If there are no ordered components, the histogram should follow a Rayleigh distribution given by

$$P(V) = \frac{V}{2\pi\sigma V^2} e^{-\frac{V^2}{2\sigma V^2}} \quad \text{for } V \geq 0$$

where $V^2 = X^2 + Y^2$ and σ_V^2, the variance of the magnitude of a phasor V, $= (2 - \pi/2)\sigma^2 = 0.42\sigma^2$. Here $\sigma^2 = <X^2> - <X>^2$. The symbol $<X>$ denotes the mean of X. It can be easily found that $<V> = 1.91\sigma_V$. This means the signal-to-noise ratio for a Rayleigh distributed signal should be a constant at 1.91.

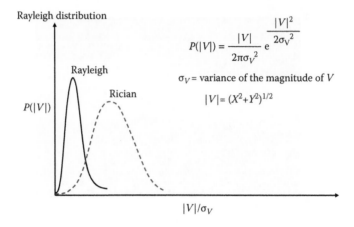

$$P(|V|) = \frac{|V|}{2\pi\sigma_V{}^2} e^{\frac{|V|^2}{2\sigma_V{}^2}}$$

σ_V = variance of the magnitude of V

$$|V| = (X^2 + Y^2)^{1/2}$$

Figure 4.18 Histograms or probability density function (PDF) of echo amplitude from biological tissues follow a Rician distribution (dashed line), a special form of which is the Rayleigh distribution (solid line). $P(V)$ is the probability density at an amplitude V and σ is the variance of V.

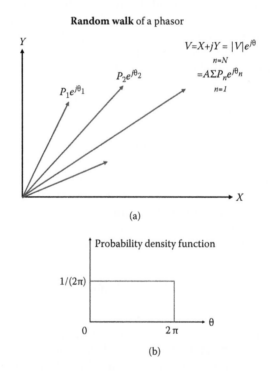

$$V = X + jY = |V|e^{j\theta}$$

$$= A\sum_{n=1}^{n=N} P_n e^{j\theta_n}$$

(a)

(b)

Figure 4.19 (a) Random walk problem of a phasor. (b) Uniformly distributed probability density function for the phase of a phasor.

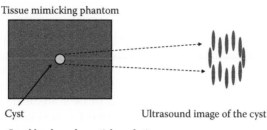

Tissue mimicking phantom

Cyst   Ultrasound image of the cyst

Speckles degrade spatial resolution

Figure 4.20 Speckles degrade spatial resolution.

The question about whether the speckle is a friend or foe has been debated for many years. On one end, speckles provide diagnostic information for the clinicians to make a diagnosis. A clear example is that different organs exhibit different speckle or textural patterns, and tumors frequently exhibit different speckle patterns from normal tissues. On the other end, speckles degrade spatial resolution of the imaging system, as illustrated in Figure 4.20. Smaller objects may be obscured by the speckles. The most optimal resolution appears to smooth out somewhat the speckle pattern while maintaining as much as possible the spatial resolution and the frame rate. Frame averaging via spatial compounding or frequency compounding has been studied and implemented in commercial scanners. Spatial or frequency compounding describes a signal processing scheme in which multiple frames are acquired either at different imaging angles or spatial positions or at different frequencies and subsequently averaged to form one frame of image. Figure 4.21 shows a thyroid image obtained with spatial compounding in which the speckle pattern is minimized.

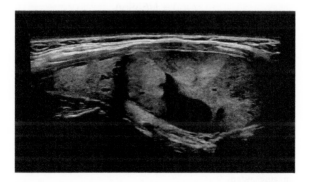

Figure 4.21 Compounded ultrasound image of a thyroid. (Courtesy of Philips Ultrasound.)

4.1.4 Image quality

Image quality may be assessed merely by observing the image in a highly subjective manner. The most objective way of assessing the image quality of an ultrasound system is to use the receiving operator characteristics (ROC) curves (Shung et al., 1992), where the human involvement is included. In order for the conclusion to be statistically meaningful, many subjects need to be studied to obtain a measurement in which both inter- and intraobserver variations are considered. Although this approach is the most desirable, it is very complicated and expensive. Simpler but quantitative measures such as spatial resolution and contrast resolution are often preferred. Spatial resolution can be assessed by imaging standardized targets or phantoms consisting of point or wire targets embedded in water or tissue-mimicking materials. Spatial resolution measured in this way depends strongly upon the instrument settings. A more convenient approach is to determine the point spread function of the system.

4.1.4.1 Point spread function

The point spread function of an imaging system (Shung et al., 1992) is the spatial point response, which is the inverse spatial Fourier transform of the spatial transfer function of an imaging system if it can be treated as a linear system, as shown in Figure 4.22. Suppose that the point spread function and the spatial transfer function of an imaging system can be denoted as $h(\mathbf{x})$ and $H(\mathbf{v})$, respectively, where $\mathbf{x}$ and $\mathbf{v}$ are vectors representing spatial distances with a unit of cm and spatial frequencies with a unit of cycles per cm. The input (the object to be imaged), S, and output (the image acquired by the imaging system), O, are related by the following equation in the spatial frequency domain:

$$O(\mathbf{v}) = H(\mathbf{v})S(\mathbf{v}) \tag{4.5}$$

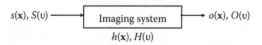

$\mathbf{x}, \mathbf{v}$: Distance in 3D, spatial frequency in 3D (cycles/cm)

$s(\mathbf{x}), S(\mathbf{v})$ = inputs in the spatial and spatial frequency domains

$o(\mathbf{x}), O(\mathbf{v})$ = outputs in the spatial and spatial frequency domains

$h(\mathbf{x}), H(\mathbf{v})$ = impulse response and transfer function of the imaging system

Figure 4.22 An imaging system is treated as a linear system.

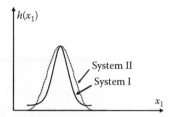

Figure 4.23 Point spread functions of two imaging systems represented by gray-scale distributions as a function of one spatial dimension. System I has a narrow point spread function, and therefore better spatial resolution than system II.

In the spatial domain their relationship is given by

$$o(\mathbf{x}) = h(\mathbf{x}) * s(\mathbf{x}) = \int_{-\infty}^{\infty} s(\mathbf{x})h(\mathbf{x}-\chi)d\chi \qquad (4.6)$$

where * denotes convolution.

The point spread function of an ultrasound system can be assessed by imaging a small point target embedded in a homogeneous gel medium or a point target suspended in a water bath and mapping the gray level of the image. Figure 4.23 shows the gray level of such an image as a function of one dimension of the spatial vector, $\mathbf{x}$, represented by x_1. System I, which has a shaper point spread function, should have a better resolution than system II. In ultrasonic imaging, the point spread function or lateral resolution is typically assessed by a wire phantom, which consists of fine wires arranged along a line embedded in a tissue-mimicking material, shown in Figure 4.24.

4.1.4.2 Contrast

Spatial resolutions of an imaging system are also affected by other parameters, including noise and the contrast of the object to be imaged. Figure 4.25 shows a spherical void with scattering property, which may be represented by η_o, the backscattering coefficient as discussed in Chapter 2, surrounded by a background medium with backscattering coefficient η_m. The object contrast may be defined as

$$\gamma_o = \frac{\eta_o - \eta_m}{\eta_0} \qquad (4.7)$$

The image contrast is defined as

$$\gamma_i = \frac{g_o - g_m}{g_0} \qquad (4.8)$$

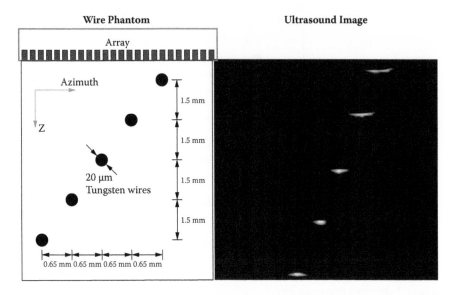

Figure 4.24 Spatial resolution of an ultrasonic imaging system is frequently assessed with a wire phantom.

where g_o and g_m denote the video signals or gray levels of the object and background. A good imaging system would enhance or accentuate the object contrast. The minimum contrast required for an imaging system to detect the object of a specific size in the presence of image noise is called contrast resolution.

These two parameters are interrelated. A system with superior resolution for high-contrast objects may not be capable of maintaining the same resolution as the contrast is reduced.

Side lobes and grating lobes produced by a single-element transducer or array, discussed in Chapter 3, are undesirable because they would cause

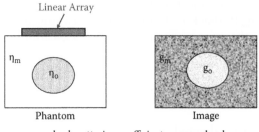

η = backscattering coefficient, g = gray level

Figure 4.25 Diagram denoting a spherical void phantom with a scattering property different from the surrounding medium and the corresponding image.

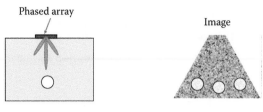

Spherical void phantom

Figure 4.26 Side lobes and grating lobes generated by arrays produce artifacts and degrade contrast resolution.

artifacts and degrade the contrast resolution of an ultrasonic imaging system. This is illustrated in Figure 4.26. There is a spherical void in the phantom. Instead of producing one image of the void, two more images are generated by the grating lobes. In addition, the echoes resulting from the side lobes or grating lobes will contribute to the echoes generated by the main lobe or beam. For a void with no scatterers, these echoes produced by the side or grating lobes will appear in the void, reducing the contrast between the void and the surrounding medium.

4.1.4.3 Noises

There are two sources for noises in an ultrasonic imaging system: acoustic noises produced by the transducer/array and spurious acoustic interactions and electronic noises produced by the imaging system itself. Acoustic noises may result from the cross talk among elements in an array and between the active element(s) and the support structures, from spurious reflections and refractions, and from grating and side lobes. The electronic noises are generated by the cross-coupling of cables and electronic components and active devices themselves. Typically acoustic noises are larger than electronic noises and more troublesome.

4.1.5 Phase aberration compensation

In commercial scanners, the sound velocity in tissues is assumed to be a constant. This could cause image degradation if the sound velocity of a region of tissues deviates substantially from this assumed value, as illustrated in Figure 4.27. It is known that fat and skin have velocities that differ appreciably from 1540 m/s. Transmitted wavefront is distorted as it propagates through skin, fat, and other tissues. Confounding this problem, the arrival times of retuned echoes are distorted again. The predetermined time delays calculated with the assumed velocity in the beamformer may not be sufficiently accurate to achieve proper focus. This issue is especially severe when imaging obese patients. Various methods have been used to compensate for this aberration caused by the phase difference of

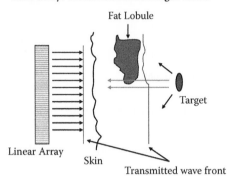

Figure 4.27 Source of phase aberration in ultrasonic imaging.

the pulses arriving at the transducers or arrays (Flax and O'Donnell, 1988; Nock and Trahey, 1989). One method uses a region of a tissue with prominent features, e.g., a blood vessel, as a target. Figure 4.28 describes how this can be achieved. The arrival times of all returned echoes at each element of an array or pulses returned from a target are adjusted via cross-correlation of the echo waveform with a reference waveform. This concept will be described in detail again in Chapter 6. Another method compensates for the velocity difference by adjusting the delays of the arriving echoes until the brightness from a region of tissues is maximized. These methods have all been demonstrated to be capable of improving image quality under certain conditions. Their capability is limited because the

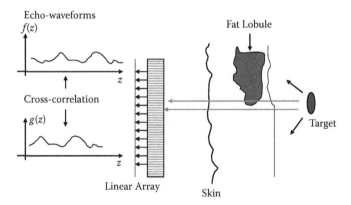

Figure 4.28 Phase aberration compensation can be carried out by cross-correlating the returned echo waveforms.

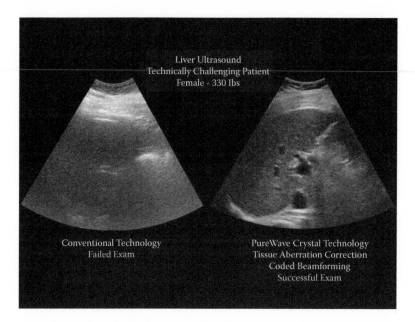

Figure 4.29 The quality of a phase aberration-compensated liver image is drastically improved. (Courtesy of Philips Ultrasound.)

phase difference in the elevational plane cannot be compensated. Further, they slow down the frame rate. These approaches may play a more significant role if phase aberration compensation is implemented on multidimensional arrays. Figure 4.29 shows the image improvement obtained with the implementation of phase aberration correction on an obese patient.

4.1.6 Clinical applications

There are numerous clinical applications of B-mode ultrasound because it is noninvasive and can display 2D cross-sectional images of anatomical structures in real time. It is used in obstetrics for monitoring the status of a fetus, in gynecology for diagnosing problems in the ovary, in general radiology for diagnosing liver tumors and gall bladder diseases, in vascular surgery for detecting arterial stenosis and deep vein thrombosis and characterizing atherosclerotic plaques, and in cardiology for diagnosing valvular diseases and monitoring the integrity of cardiac wall functions, to name just a few.

4.2 M-mode and C-mode

In M-mode display, one intensity-modulated A-line or B-line is swept across the monitor as a function of time at a rate much slower than the pulse repetition frequency (PRF) of the A-line, as illustrated in Figure 4.30.

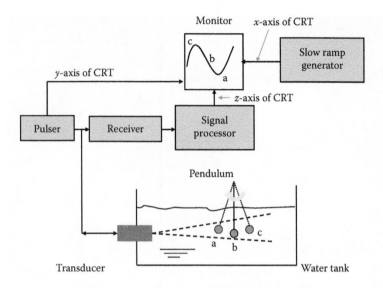

Figure 4.30 Block diagram of an M-mode ultrasonic imaging system.

The sweep of the electron beam in the x-axis is controlled by a slow ramp generator, whereas the triggering of the y-axis is synchronized with the pulser. The rest of the device is similar to the A-mode. In this format, the ultrasound beam is fixed at a certain position or angle and the displacement of a target relative to the probe along the beam direction is displayed as a function of time. The motion of a swinging pendulum at positions a, b, and c can be clearly discerned on the display. This type of display is most useful for monitoring the motion of anatomical structure, for example, valves in the heart. Figure 4.31 shows the M-mode display of a mitral valve prolapse, an abnormal displacement of the valvular leaflets. Needless to say, in current scanners M-mode is easily implemented digitally and is an option mostly used for cardiac scanning.

C-mode is a form of display similar to conventional radiography if a second transducer is used to detect the pulse after traversing a medium, illustrated in Figure 4.32. The image obtained is then a 2D gray-scale map of the ultrasonic attenuation coefficient experienced by the pulse in the object. Reflection-type C-mode ultrasonography is also possible by time gating the returned echoes to select only those that originate from a certain plane or at a constant depth relative to the transducer, as illustrated in Figure 4.33. The concept of time gating is described in Figure 4.34. The time gate is primarily a switch that is turned on by an external pulse and lets the input waveform pass. The output signal consists of only the input waveform within the time duration in which the gate is on. C-mode display is not used often in clinical scanners, but is quite popular in acoustic

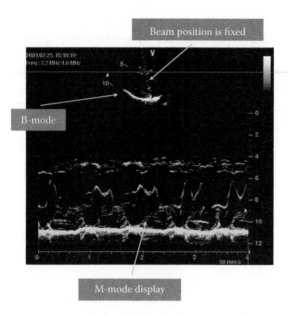

Figure 4.31 M-mode image of a mitral valve. The top of the figure is a B-mode display of the heart. The white line indicates the ultrasound beam direction along which the M-mode image in the bottom is acquired. (Courtesy of GE Medical Systems.)

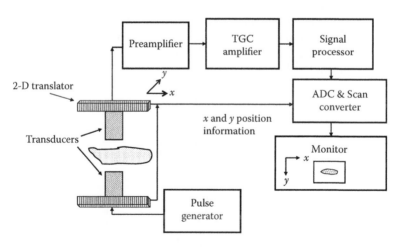

Figure 4.32 Block diagram of a C-mode ultrasonic imaging system for obtaining an attenuation map.

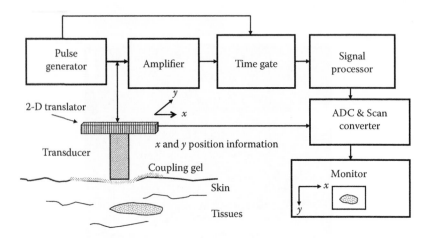

Figure 4.33 Block diagram of a C-mode ultrasonic imaging system for making a reflection (scattering) map.

microscopy that can be operated either in B-mode or in C-mode at frequencies ranging from 40 MHz to 3 GHz. Acoustic microscopy has many applications in nondestructive evaluation of materials, such as integrated circuits, but is of only limited interest in biomedicine.

4.3 Ultrasound computed tomography (CT)

Computed tomography has been successfully used in x-ray and magnetic resonance imaging to produce tomograms defined as 2D images of 2D slices. The CT principle is quite straightforward and can easily be implemented once the signals are digitized so that they can be processed with a computer (Shung et al., 1992). For CT reconstruction, a 2D object of interest

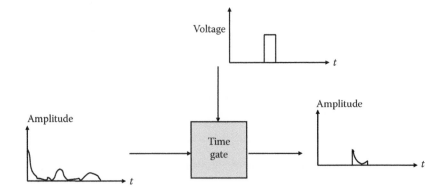

Figure 4.34 Time gate performs the function of turning on and off a signal in time.

is divided into many pixels or voxels in 3D. The property of the pixel can be retrieved by performing multiple measurements at different positions or angles with the imaging system. For x-ray CT, x-ray generators and detectors are used to perform such measurements to estimate the x-ray attenuation coefficients of all pixels. An image is formed from mapping the estimated attenuation coefficient to a gray scale. It is plausible that the CT principle can be readily extended to ultrasound. The feasibility of ultrasound CT has been studied for many years (Greenleaf, 1983). Two types of ultrasound CT images (attenuation CT and velocity CT) can be obtained since ultrasound propagation in a tissue is affected by attenuation and sound velocity. The difference lies in that in one, the ultrasound property in a pixel to be estimated is sound velocity, whereas in the other, attenuation is estimated. A graphical illustration of ultrasound attenuation CT is shown in Figure 4.35. One transducer is used as a transmitter, whereas the other is used as a receiver. For the sake of simplicity, the object of interest is divided only into four pixels, each assigned an intensity attenuation coefficient denoted by $\beta = 2\alpha$. The pixel dimensions are represented by Δx and Δy. The transmitted intensities are exponentially related to the incident intensity, as discussed in Chapter 2. The transmitter and receiver assembly is translated and then rotated to collect multiple sets of data. In Figure 4.35, only four sets of data are shown. The data sets are inverted to extract the ultrasound properties assuming that Δx and Δy are equal (this is a valid assumption when the number of pixels is large). Mathematical iteration among a host of methods has been used to accomplish the data inversion (Shung et al., 1992). Ultrasound CT has achieved limited success to date. The reason is twofold. First, the ultrasound beam cannot be approximated as a pencil beam because it is refracted as it

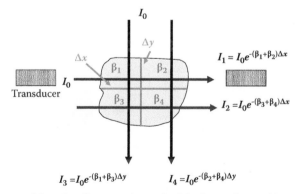

More than four equations solved for four unknown β's

Figure 4.35 Graphical illustration of ultrasound CT principle. β = intensity attenuation coefficient = 2α.

propagates through an interface. In addition, it suffers losses not only due to attenuation, but also due to reflection at tissue interfaces and beam diffraction. Second, ultrasound cannot penetrate into regions of the body that contain bones and air. Even so, ultrasound CT has been envisioned to have potential applications in imaging organs like breast and testicles. Although sophisticated mathematical algorithms have been developed to solve the so-called inverse problem, i.e., extracting the pixel value from the data obtained or projections, thus far only limited success has been achieved. The image quality is inferior to B-mode images and also contains undesirable computational artifacts.

4.4 *Coded excitation imaging*

The instantaneous intensity of the transmitted pulse and the energy contained in the pulse is regulated by the Food and Drug Administration (FDA) and is thus limited because of the concern with potential bioeffects. As a result, although it is known that increasing the pulse energy will increase the signal-to-noise ratio of the returned echoes, this simply cannot be done and is not a valid alternative in biomedical imaging. Several scanner manufacturers have adopted a novel approach to overcome this limitation, in which the increased energy is spread over a longer time duration while maintaining the instantaneous intensity level. This form of imaging uses a transmitted signal consisting of a frequency modulated chirp or a series of binary coded pulses, shown in Figure 4.36 (O'Donnell, 1992). The returned echoes are matched with the excitation signals to retrieve the pulse amplitude. As illustrated in Figure 4.37, there are two different types of binary codes: one requiring a single transmission and another requiring multiple transmissions. Figure 4.38(a) and (b) shows, respectively, a chirped signal and a Barker coded signal. The number 13 means that the code consists of 13 pulses.

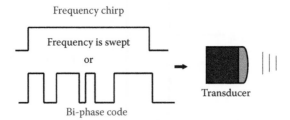

Figure 4.36 Excitation signals to the transducer of an ultrasonic imaging system may be encoded by frequency or pulse duration. The resulting benefit is the increased ultrasonic energy imparted into the body because of the longer exposure duration, and thus the improved signal-to-noise ratio and increased depth of penetration.

	Single - Tx	Multiple-Tx
Phase coding	Barker	Golay
Frequency coding	Chirp	

Figure 4.37 Different types of codes have been used for coded excitation.

Figure 4.39, where one box represents one sinusoidal cycle, shows that for uncoded signal, its autocorrelation achieves the highest signal-to-noise ratio (a), whereas for the Barker coded signal, its cross-correlation with the matched decoding filter yields an output of the same peak and yet much reduced range side lobes. The Golay codes, which require two

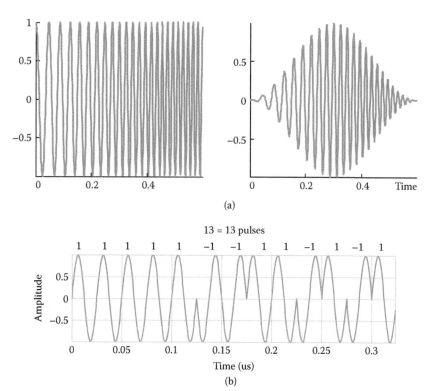

Figure 4.38 (a) A chirped signal. (b) A biphasic coded signal.

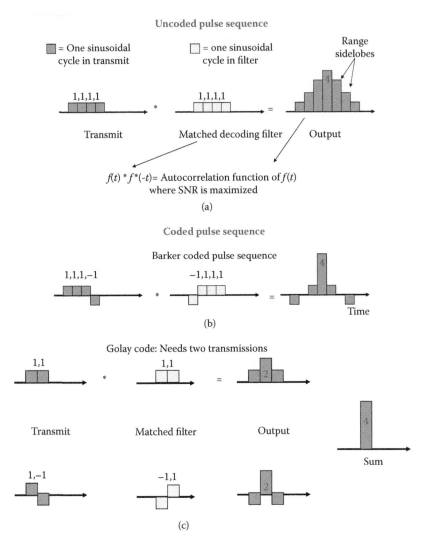

Figure 4.39 A comparison of (a) uncoded signal, (b) Barker coded signal, and (c) Golay coded signal in performance.

transmissions, outperform the Barker codes (Figure 4.39(c)). Figure 4.40 gives an example on how the coding works. Two coded waveforms are cross-correlated to produce the output waveform in the bottom. Figure 4.41 shows that bi-phasic code outperforms the chirp code with a smaller-range lobe.

The benefit of coded excitation imaging is the increased depth of penetration at the cost of increased complexity, reduced frame rate, and slightly

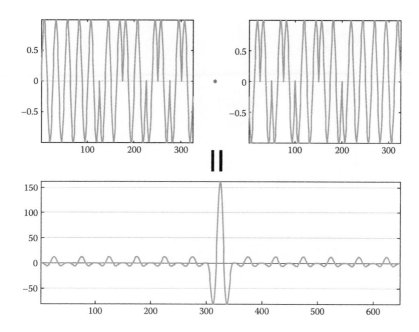

Figure 4.40 Actual implementation of Barker coded signal processing.

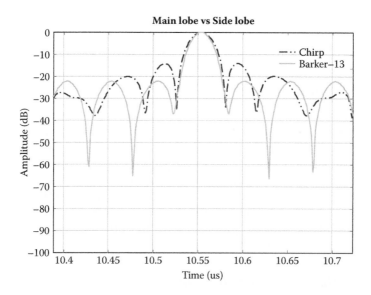

Figure 4.41 A comparison of performance of chirped and Barker coded signal processing.

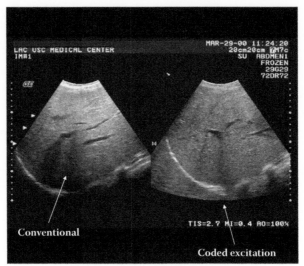

7 MHz, 20 cm depth of penetration

Figure 4.42 A comparison of B-mode and coded excitation image of liver. (Courtesy of GE Medical Systems.)

inferior axial resolution. These problems have now been largely overcome. Demonstrated in Figure 4.42, the quality of coded excitation image is comparable to that of conventional B-mode image, but with increased depth of penetration, which is beneficial in imaging obese patients.

4.5 Compound imaging

As was discussed in previous sections, compound scan can suppress speckle pattern, improving contrast and image quality at a cost of reduced scanning speed. During the time when static scanners were the workhorse, this was indeed a problem. Increased speed in electronics and computer processing has allowed compound scanning to be achieved in real time with linear arrays. The beam is electronically steered into multiple directions and images are superimposed. The superior image quality resulting from compounding is apparent. An image obtained with compound imaging is shown in Figure 4.21.

4.6 Synthetic aperture imaging

In order to reduce the cost in beamforming for arrays where hundreds of electronic channels are needed, synthetic aperture imaging can be used (Karaman and O'Donnell, 1995). Synthetic aperture imaging can be

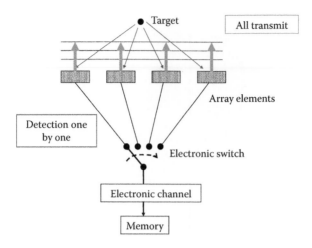

Figure 4.43 Synthetic aperture imaging during reception.

accomplished in receive only or in both transmit and receive. Synthetic aperture imaging during receive is illustrated in Figure 4.43, where only four linear elements are shown. All four elements are excited simultaneously for transmission to achieve the largest aperture that is required to obtain the best lateral resolution. During reception, a switch is used to sample the waveform detected at each element, so that only one channel of electronics is needed, in contrast to conventional imaging, where four channels are needed. The data from all elements can be stored in a memory for later processing, which includes applying the delays for focusing, filtering, and scan conversion. Its advantage is the reduced cost and complexity, which are important in such cases as intravascular imaging, where the disposable probe is so small that it is impossible to mount a large number of integrated circuits in the probe.

4.7 New developments

For high-end ultrasonic imaging systems, more options are constantly added. Elasticity imaging is one of them. Harmonic imaging in conjunction with the injection of contrast agent is another. Both will be discussed in detail in later chapters. There is, however, a trend toward miniaturization of the system to make it more portable and easier to use. A great application for this type of scanners is in emergency medicine. A number of manufacturers have successfully entered this market. Figure 4.44 shows portable scanners made by (1) Fuji Sonoite, (2) Siemens, and (3) GE. They all have very simple functions and are capable of color Doppler imaging, which will be discussed in Chapter 5. The GE Vscan pocket scanner weighs only 390 g.

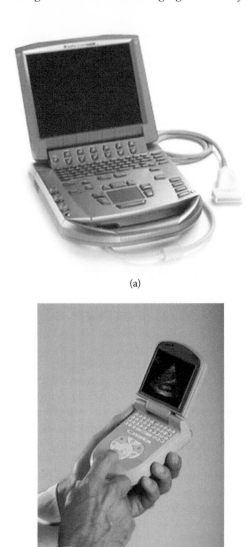

(a)

(b)

Figure 4.44 Portable scanners from three different manufacturers: (a) Fuji Sonosite (courtesy of Sonosite), (b) pocket scanner with a 3 MHz element-phased array (courtesy of Siemens), and (c) Vscan phased array system with color Doppler (courtesy of GE).

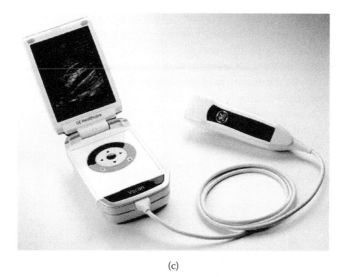

(c)

Figure 4.44 *(Continued)* Portable scanners from three different manufacturers: (a) Fuji Sonosite (courtesy of Sonosite), (b) pocket scanner with a 3 MHz element-phased array (courtesy of Siemens), and (c) Vscan phased array system with color Doppler (courtesy of GE).

Another advancement is the elimination of the cable that connects an ultrasonic probe to the imaging console by adopting wireless technology. Figure 4.45 shows a wireless portable scanner developed by Siemens where the wireless radio frequency (RF) signal is transmitted at 8.7 GHz.

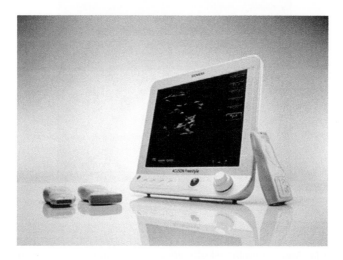

Figure 4.45 A wireless scanner capable of color Doppler. (Courtesy of Siemens.)

Although ultrasound computed tomographical scanners have only found limited success in breast imaging, a new breast scanner very similar to x-ray mammography has recently been introduced. A unique feature of this scanner is the concave curved linear array probe that conforms better to the breast curvature. The linear array is mechanically scanned linearly to acquire multiple slices of B-mode images for later 3D reconstruction. It was approved by the FDA for dense breast scanning as a complementary tool for x-ray mammography. Figure 4.46(a) shows how the

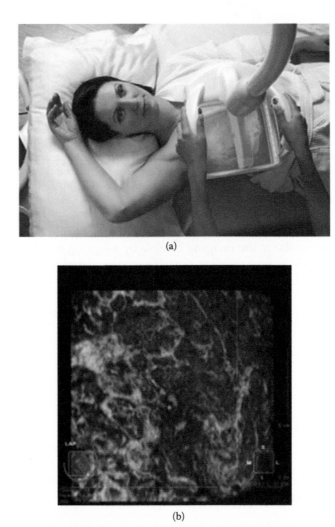

(a)

(b)

Figure 4.46 (a) Automated breast ultrasonic scanner and (b) corresponding coronal image. (Courtesy of GE.)

linear mechanical scanning of the linear array is performed on a patient
and (b) a coronal B-mode breast image acquired by such a scanner, which
shows a lesion at the lower right-hand corner. A coronal view, which is not
possible with a conventional ultrasound scanner, can be obtained following 3D reconstruction.

References and Further Reading Materials

Flax SW and O'Donnell M. Phase-aberration correction using signals from point
    reflectors and diffuse scatterers: Basic principles. *IEEE Trans Ultrasonics
    Ferroelect Freq Cont* 1988; 35: 768–778.
Greenleaf JF. Computerized tomography with ultrasound. *Proc IEEE* 1983; 71:
    330–337.
Karaman M and O'Donnell M. Synthetic aperture imaging for small scale systems.
    IEEE Trans Ultrasonics Ferroelect Freq Cont 1995; 42: 429–442.
Nock L and Trahey GE. Phase aberration correction in medical ultrasound using
    speckle brightness as a quality factor. *J Acoust Soc Am* 1989; 85: 1819–1826.
O'Donnell M. Coded excitation system for improving the penetration of real-time
    phased array imaging system. *IEEE Trans Ultrasonics Ferroelect Freq Cont*
    1992; 39: 341–351.
Ophir J and Maklad NF. Digital scan converters in diagnostic ultrasound imaging.
    Proceedings of the IEEE 1979; 67: 654–664.
Shung KK, Smith MB, and Tui BWN. *Principles of medical imaging.* San Diego:
    Academic Press, 1992.
Shung KK and Thieme GA. *Ultrasonic scattering by biological tissues.* Boca Raton,
    FL: CRC Press, 1993.
Thomenius KE. Evolution of ultrasound beamformers. In Levy M, Schneider SC,
    and McVoy BR (eds.), *Proceedings of the 1996 IEEE Ultrasonics Symposium,*
    New York, 1996, pp. 1615–1622.
Wagner RF, Smith SW, Sandrik JM, and Lopez H. Statistics of speckle in ultrasound
    B-scans. *IEEE Trans Soncis Ultrasonics* 1983; 30: 156–163.

chapter five

Doppler flow measurements

As was discussed earlier in Chapter 2, the Doppler effect provides a unique capability for ultrasound to measure blood flow (Evans and McDicken, 2000; Jensen, 1996). Upon insonification by an ultrasound beam, the echoes scattered by blood carry information about the velocity of blood flow. Blood flow measurements are frequently performed in a clinical environment to assess the state of blood vessels and functions of an organ. Ultrasonic Doppler instruments allow a measurement of instantaneous blood flow velocity. Combined with pulse-echo instruments, instantaneous flow rate in a blood vessel as a function of time and cardiac output can be measured noninvasively with ultrasound. At present, very few clinical options are available to do so. Figure 5.1 shows an ultrasound beam of frequency f insonifying a blood vessel, making an angle of θ relative to the velocity v. Here it is assumed that blood flows in a vessel with a uniform velocity v. The returned echoes are Doppler shifted. The Doppler shift frequency f_d is related to the ultrasound frequency f by Equation (2.43):

$$f_d = \frac{2v\cos\theta}{c}f$$

where c is the sound velocity in blood and may be assumed to be 1540 m/s. The Doppler-shifted frequencies happen to be in the audio range for blood flow velocities in the human body for an ultrasound frequency between 1 to 15 MHz.

Conventionally, two different approaches have been used for ultrasonic Doppler flow measurements: continuous-wave (CW) and pulsed-wave (PW) Doppler.

5.1 Nondirectional CW flowmeters

A CW system is shown in Figure 5.2. A probe consisting of two piezoelectric elements, one for transmitting the ultrasound signal and one for receiving echoes returned from blood, is excited by an oscillator. The Doppler-shifted echoes are amplified, demodulated, and band pass filtered to remove the carrier frequency and other spurious signals. Suppose that the ultrasound signal generated by the oscillator is given by

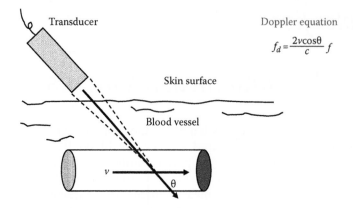

Figure 5.1 An ultrasound beam is incident upon a blood vessel and makes an angle of θ relative to the direction of blood flow.

$A\cos(\omega t)$, where A denotes signal amplitude and ω (the angular frequency) $= 2\pi f$. The demodulated signal would be

$$g_d(\omega,\omega_d) = A\cos(\omega t)B\cos[(\omega+\omega_d)t] = \frac{1}{2}AB\{\cos[(2\omega+\omega_d)t]+\cos(\omega_d t)\}$$

where the echoes are represented by $B\cos[(\omega + \omega_d)t]$ and $\omega_d = 2\pi f_d$. The magnitude of constant B is determined by the scattering strength of blood. Much work has been done to better understand the relationship between the Doppler power generated by blood and hematological

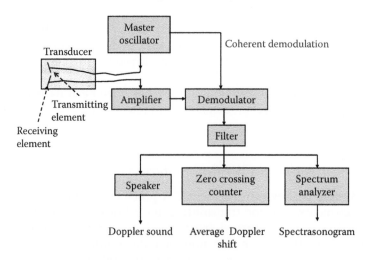

Figure 5.2 Block diagram of a CW Doppler flowmeter.

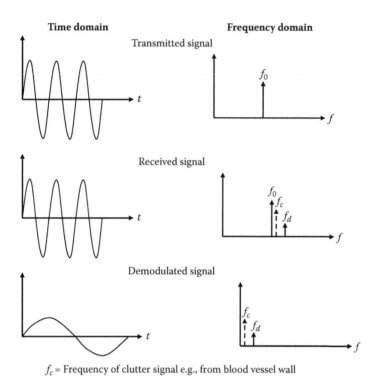

f_c = Frequency of clutter signal e.g., from blood vessel wall

Figure 5.3 Doppler signals in the time and frequency domain showing the effect of demodulation.

and hemodynamic factors (Shung et al., 1992; Mo and Cobbold, 1993). Doppler power from blood has been found to be related to flow disturbance, hematocrit, and the degree of red blood aggregation, which is in turn affected by the concentration of plasma proteins such as fibrinogen and local shear rate. The output of the demodulator contains both the ultrasound carrier frequency and the Doppler shift, illustrated in Figure 5.3, where the signals in the time and frequency domains are shown, respectively, on the left and right. The carrier signal can be readily removed by band pass filtering by setting the cutoff frequency of the band pass filter at the high end to be much lower than the carrier frequency. A problem in ultrasonic Doppler blood flow measurement is that the blood vessels that produce large reflected echoes are slow moving as well. In Doppler terminology, these large, slow-moving echoes are called clutter signals, shown in Figure 5.3 as f_c. The cutoff frequency of the band pass filter at the low end has to be designed to minimize the interference of these clutter signals. The design of this band pass filter in the low-frequency region, which performs the function of high pass,

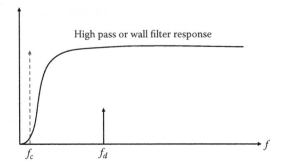

Figure 5.4 Clutter rejection filter or wall filter is used to suppress large echoes produced by slow-moving blood vessel walls. f_c = frequency of clutter signal (e.g., from blood vessel wall).

also called clutter rejection filter, has been problematic due to the fact that the magnitude of clutter signals is several orders higher than those from blood and may mask those from slow-moving blood (Figure 5.4). A filter with a very steep slope or a method that carries out some forms of echo cancellation may be used (Jensen, 1996). The signal after band-pass filtering can be processed in different ways. It may be heard with a speaker since the Doppler shift is in the audible range. Alternatively, a zero-crossing counter can be used to estimate the mean Doppler frequency, or a spectrum analyzer can be used to display the spectrum. The zero-crossing counter estimates the number of zero-crossings of a signal. The number of zero-crossings, N, and the mean frequency, f_m, of a signal are given, respectively, by

$$N = 2\sqrt{\frac{\int_0^\infty f^2 P(f)\,df}{\int_0^\infty P(f)\,df}} \tag{5.1}$$

$$f_m = \frac{\int_0^\infty f P(f)\,df}{\int_0^\infty P(f)\,df} \tag{5.2}$$

where $P(f)$ is the probability density function at frequency f. For a pure sinusoidal signal of frequency f_m, $N = 2f_m$. Complication arises if the signal is not sinusoidal, as in the case of Doppler flow measurements, where

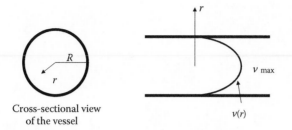

Figure 5.5 Laminar blood flow in an artery has a parabolic flow profile.

the blood flow is not uniform. For blood flow in a vessel, the velocity is related to radial distance r, shown in Figure 5.5, by the following equation (Nichols and O'Rourke, 1990):

$$v(r) = v_{max} \left[1 - \left(\frac{r}{R} \right)^n \right] \tag{5.3}$$

where v_{max} is the peak velocity, n is an index indicating the nature of flow, and R is the radius of the blood vessel. For parabolic flow, $n = 2$ and $N = 1.15 f_{max}$, where f_{max} is the maximal Doppler frequency.

The spectrum is usually displayed in the format shown in Figure 5.6(a), where the vertical axis indicates Doppler frequency or velocity, the horizontal axis indicates time, and the gray scale indicates the intensity of the Doppler signal at that frequency or velocity. Figure 5.6(b) illustrates how one vertical line in the Doppler sonogram is calculated and the complete Doppler sonogram obtained. At each instant of time, the vertical line displayed represents the Doppler spectrum calculated at that time within a 5 to 10 ms time window. For a timescale of many seconds, the Doppler spectrum obtained within a very short window at a certain time can be represented by a line. From the Doppler spectrum, the mean frequency or other frequencies, e.g., median frequency, where the Doppler power spectrum is split into two equal halves, and mode frequency, where the Doppler power is the highest, can be readily estimated.

Doppler flowmeters have been used to noninvasively assess vascular disorders. Flow disturbances near a stenosis cause the Doppler spectrum to broaden because blood flow velocity fluctuates. There is, however, a caveat that must be recognized to avoid misdiagnoses: transit time spectral broadening. This is illustrated in Figure 5.7(a) for a single scatterer traversing an ultrasound beam at velocity v. A finite time is needed for the scatterer to traverse the beam. In the time domain, there is a finite time duration, which is defined by Δt (–3 dB time duration from peak value),

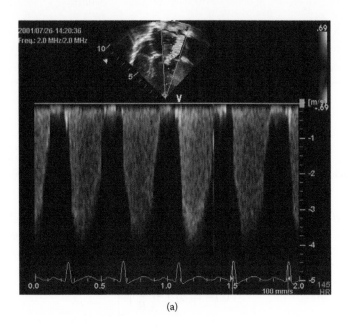

(a)

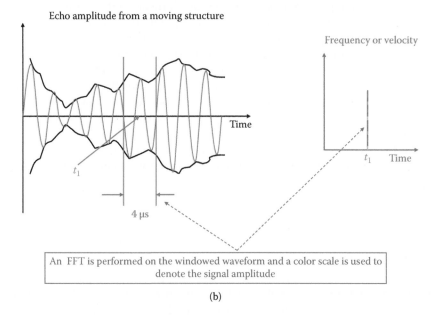

An FFT is performed on the windowed waveform and a color scale is used to denote the signal amplitude

(b)

Figure 5.6 (a) Spectrasonogram of CW Doppler signals produced by a mitral valve regurgitation jet. The top image is a B-mode apical four-chamber view of the heart. The dotted line indicates the direction of the Doppler beam. (Courtesy of GE Medical Systems.) (b) How a spectrasonogram is calculated.

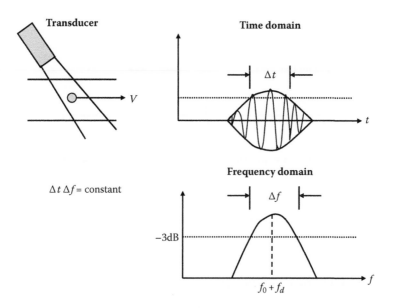

Figure 5.7 Transit time broadening causes an increase in the bandwidth in the frequency domain of the Doppler spectrum.

shown in Figure 5.7(b). Translated into the frequency domain, the result is a spectrum with a bandwidth Δf purely caused by this transit time effect, instead of a single Doppler spectral line representing velocity v. This is graphically displayed in Figure 5.7(c).

5.2 Directional Doppler flowmeters

Nondirectional Doppler devices cannot differentiate the direction of blood flow. A few methods have been developed to extract flow direction from the Doppler signal.

5.2.1 Single-sideband filtering

In Figure 5.2, it is possible to divide the output from the demodulator into two paths. In one path, a high-pass filter is used to filter out signals at frequencies lower than f_0, whereas in the other a low-pass filter is used to filter out signals higher than f_0, as illustrated in Figure 5.8. In Figure 5.8 the portions of the spectrum above and below f_0 are, respectively, the forward flow and reverse flow Doppler signals. In this way, the output from one channel contains only forward flow signals and the other, reverse flow signals. Although this approach is straightforward, the design of the

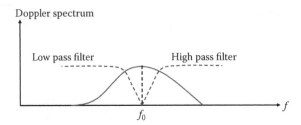

Figure 5.8 Two filters around the carrier frequency can be used to separate forward and reverse flow.

filters can be difficult because the drop-off regions of these filters are very close to f_0.

5.2.2 Heterodyne demodulation

The block diagram of a directional Doppler device that uses heterodyne demodulation is given in Figure 5.9. A heterodyne oscillator generates a sinusoidal signal at a frequency f_h. The mixer between the oscillator and the heterodyne oscillator performs a multiplication operation. Its output is given by

$$g_{m1}(\omega_0,\omega_h) = C\cos(\omega_0 t)D\cos(\omega_h t) = \frac{1}{2}CD[\cos(\omega_0 + \omega_h)t + \cos(\omega_0 - \omega_h)t]$$

where C and D are the amplitudes of the signals produced by the oscillator and the heterodyne oscillator, respectively. For the sake of simplicity, assume that $C = D = 1$ because here only the frequencies are of concern. After low-pass filtering, only the $\cos(\omega_0 - \omega_h)t$ term is left. This signal is then mixed again with the signals detected by the receiving transducer element that contains the Doppler-shifted frequencies in both the

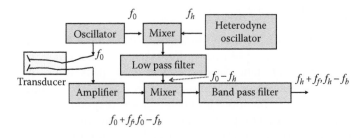

Figure 5.9 Block diagram for heterodyne demodulation. f = forward, b = backward.

forward and backward directions, $f_0 - f_b$ and $f_0 + f_f$. The output of the second mixer is

$$g_{m2}(\omega_0, \omega_h, \omega_f, \omega_b) = \cos(\omega_0 - \omega_h)t \cdot [\cos(\omega_0 + \omega_f)t + \cos(\omega_0 - \omega_b)t]$$

$$= \frac{1}{2}[\cos(2\omega_0 - \omega_h + \omega_f)t + \cos(2\omega_0 - \omega_b - \omega_h)t$$

$$+ \cos(\omega_h + \omega_f)t + \cos(\omega_h - \omega_b)t]$$

After band pass filtering, the signal becomes

$$g_d(\omega_b, \omega_f, \omega_h) = [\cos(\omega_h + \omega_f)t + \cos(\omega_h - \omega_b)t]$$

The effect of heterodyne demodulation in comparison to conventional demodulation in the frequency domain is shown in Figure 5.10.

5.2.3 Quadrature phase demodulation

Figures 5.11 and 5.12 show how quadrature phase demodulation can be used to obtain directional information. Here it is assumed again that the amplitudes of signals are all equal to 1 to simplify the mathematical operation. The direct channel output is

$$\cos \omega_0 t \cdot [\cos(\omega_0 + \omega_f)t + \cos(\omega_0 - \omega_b)t] = \frac{1}{2}[\cos(2\omega_0 + \omega_f)t + \cos(2\omega_0 - \omega_b)t$$

$$+ \cos \omega_f t + \cos \omega_b t]$$

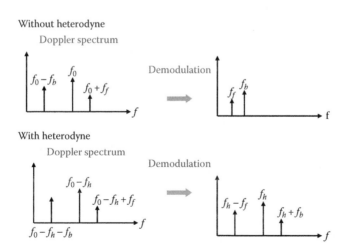

Without heterodyne
Doppler spectrum

$f_0 - f_b$ f_0
$f_0 + f_f$

$\xrightarrow{f}$

Demodulation

f_f f_b

$\xrightarrow{f}$

With heterodyne
Doppler spectrum

$f_0 - f_h$
$f_0 - f_h + f_f$

$f_0 - f_h - f_b$

$\xrightarrow{f}$

Demodulation

$f_h - f_f$ f_h
$f_h + f_b$

$\xrightarrow{f}$

Figure 5.10 The effect of heterodyne demodulation in the frequency domain.

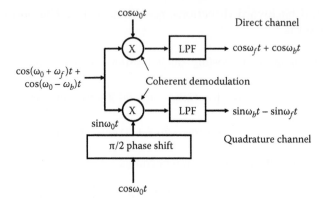

Figure 5.11 Quadrature demodulation.

After band pass filtering, the signal becomes $\cos \omega_f t + \cos \omega_b t$.
The quadrature channel output is

$$\cos\left(\omega_0 - \frac{\pi}{2}\right)t \cdot [\cos(\omega_0 + \omega_f)t + \cos(\omega_0 - \omega_b)t] = \sin \omega_0 t[\cos(\omega_0 + \omega_f)t$$

$$+ \cos(\omega_0 - \omega_b)t]$$

After low-pass filtering, the signal becomes $-\sin \omega_f t + \sin \omega_b t$.

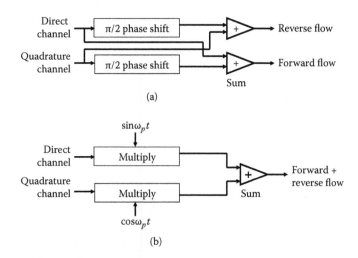

Figure 5.12 Separation of forward and reverse flows can be accomplished either (a) in the phase domain or (b) in the frequency domain.

To retrieve the directional information from these signals, a phase domain method and a frequency domain method may be used, illustrated in Figure 5.12(a) and (b), respectively. In the phase domain method, the direct channel output is summed with the quadrature channel output after $\pi/2$ phase shift to yield the forward flow signal.

$$D(t) + Q(t - \pi/2) = \cos \omega_f t + \cos \omega_b t - \sin\left(\omega_f t - \frac{\pi}{2}\right) + \sin\left(\omega_b t - \frac{\pi}{2}\right)$$

$$= 2 \cos \omega_f t$$

The direct channel output after $\pi/2$ phase shift is summed with the quadrature channel output to yield the reverse flow signal $2 \sin \omega_b t$.

In the frequency domain method, the direct channel signal is multiplied with a sinusoidal signal $\sin \omega_p t$ and summed up with the quadrature channel signal multiplied by $\cos \omega_p t$:

$$D(t) \sin \omega_p t = \sin \omega_p t \cdot [\cos \omega_f t + \cos \omega_b t]$$

$$= \frac{1}{2} [\sin(\omega_p - \omega_f)t + \sin(\omega_p + \omega_f)t + \sin(\omega_p - \omega_b)t + \sin(\omega_p + \omega_b)t]$$

$$Q(t) con \omega_p t = \cos \omega_p t \cdot [-\sin \omega_f t + \sin \omega_b t]$$

$$= \frac{1}{2} [\sin(\omega_p - \omega_f)t - \sin(\omega_p + \omega_f)t - \sin(\omega_p - \omega_b)t + \sin(\omega_p + \omega_b)t]$$

Therefore,

$$D(t) \sin \omega_p t + Q(t) con \omega_p t = \sin(\omega_p - \omega_f)t + \sin(\omega_p + \omega_b)t$$

5.3 Pulsed Doppler flowmeters

A problem with a CW Doppler is its inability to differentiate the origins of the Doppler signals produced within the ultrasound beam. Signals coming from blood flowing in two blood vessels in the same vicinity, e.g., an artery and a vein, may overlap. To alleviate this problem, a pulsed-wave Doppler may be used. As illustrated in Figure 5.13, ultrasound bursts of relatively long duration consisting of many cycles are used to excite the probe. The returned echoes received by the same transducer are amplified and demodulated. The demodulated signal is then sampled and held by a sample-and-hold circuit, which is triggered by the delayed pulses. The time-delayed pulses allow the selection of the location where the

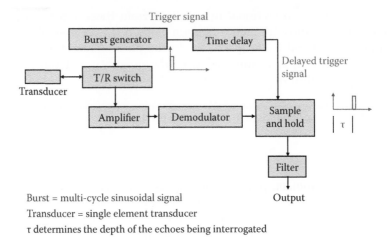

Burst = multi-cycle sinusoidal signal

Transducer = single element transducer

τ determines the depth of the echoes being interrogated

Figure 5.13 Block diagram of pulsed Doppler flowmeter.

Doppler shift frequency is monitored. Figure 5.14 illustrates the principle behind pulsed Doppler flowmeters. Each waveform in the left panel of Figure 5.14(a) represents the echo waveform received by the transducer after a burst is transmitted. The waveforms are separated by the pulse repetition period (PRP). The time delay is set to allow the sampling of the waveform at points a, b, c, d, and e. The sample-and-hold circuit samples the waveforms at these points and holds the voltage at the sampled level until the next sampling time, as illustrated in the right panel. What a pulsed Doppler flowmeter does, as illustrated in Figure 5.14(b), is to reconstruct the time waveform represented by the dashed line from discretely sampled data points separated by one pulse repetition period. Following band pass filtering, the Doppler signal can be displayed or heard as the CW Doppler.

A drawback of the pulsed Doppler is the limit of the highest Doppler frequency or maximal velocity that it can measure. This is determined by the pulse repetition frequency (PRF) of the device, which has to be at least twice as large as the maximal Doppler frequency. This may pose a problem when measuring high velocities in the body, e.g., outflow tracts of cardiac valves and stenosis in a blood vessel. To avoid aliasing, the PRF of the pulsed Doppler device has to be

$$PRF > 2f_{max}$$

$$\therefore PRF > (4v_{max}f)/c \tag{5.4}$$

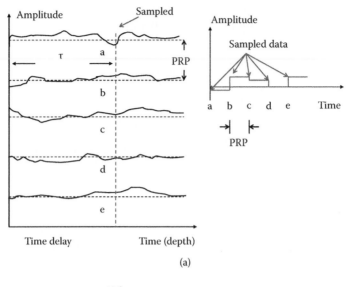

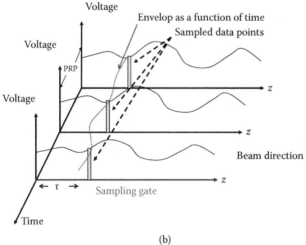

Figure 5.14 Principle used by pulsed Doppler to acquire Doppler signals: (a) sample and hold, (b) sampled data points separated by one pulse repetition period.

where f_{max} and v_{max} are, respectively, the maximal Doppler shift frequency and maximal velocity. To avoid range ambiguity, all echoes must be received before the next burst is transmitted, i.e.,

$$PRP = \frac{1}{PRF} > \frac{2z_{max}}{c} \qquad (5.5)$$

where z_{max} is the maximal depth of penetration and PRP is the pulse repetition period. Combining Equations (5.4) and (5.5),

$$v_{max} \cdot z_{max} \leq \frac{c^2}{8f} \tag{5.6}$$

The term on the right of the equation is a constant. This means that the performance of the pulsed Doppler device is limited by the maximal velocity that it can detect or the maximal depth of penetration. To enhance one, the performance of the other must be compromised. Modern high-end ultrasonic imaging machines are equipped with both CW and PW capabilities.

5.4 Clinical applications and Doppler indices

Ultrasonic Doppler devices are inexpensive and are capable of yielding clinically useful information noninvasively. Their primary applications have been in assessing cardiovascular systems, e.g., diagnosing stenosis in blood vessels and cardiac valvular diseases. They have also been used to estimate cardiac valvular stenosis (Feigenbaum, 1986). Since the velocity measured by the Doppler devices is dependent upon the Doppler angle, which is difficult to estimate, a few indices that are not angle dependent have been used frequently in a clinical setting to derive useful diagnostic data. Figure 5.15 shows the mean velocity waveform from a peripheral artery obtained with a CW Doppler flowmeter. The pulsatility index is defined as the ratio of $(S - D)/M$, where S, D, and M are the peak, minimal, and mean velocities. In this expression the angle dependence is eliminated. The pulsatility index has been found to be related to the resistance of the vessel downstream from the

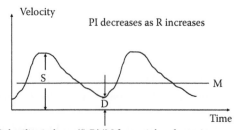

Pulsatility index = (S-D)/M for peripheral arteries
Pourcelot's index = (S-D)/S for carotid arteries
Indices are related to flow resistance i.e., downstream stenosis

Figure 5.15 Mean velocity waveform acquired with a CW flowmeter from a peripheral blood vessel can be used to derive indices useful for diagnosing vascular diseases.

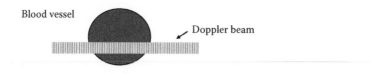

Figure 5.16 Doppler beam is smaller than the blood vessel being interrogated.

measurement site. For instance, stenosis of a downstream vessel may cause the flow resistance upstream to increase. Another useful index is the Purcelot resistance index for the carotid artery, which is defined as $(S - D)/S$.

5.5 Potential problems in Doppler measurements

In Doppler flow measurements, preventive measures must be taken to avoid errors that may result from the following problems: (1) erroneous Doppler angle estimation; (2) nonuniform insonification of vessel by the ultrasound beam, as illustrated in Figure 5.16, resulting in an erroneous estimation of the velocity; (3) aliasing of Doppler frequency estimation; (4) intrinsic spectral broadening; (5) attenuation of intervening tissues between the probe and the region of interest; and (6) clutter signals generated by slow-moving large anatomical structures. The Doppler angle can be better estimated with the aid of B-mode imaging, although it is still not ideal because of the tortuosity of blood vessels. If the sensitive volume of the ultrasound beam or beams is smaller than the vessel, portions of the blood will not be included in the measurement, resulting in estimated velocity values potentially deviating from the true values. Since the attenuation of tissues is linearly proportional to frequency, the Doppler spectrum may be affected if deeper tissues are interrogated. Other problems have been addressed in the preceding sections.

5.6 Tissue doppler and multigate Doppler

In the Doppler signal processing chain shown in Figures 5.2 and 5.13, if only large-amplitude echoes of lower Doppler frequencies from tissues such as myocardium or heart muscle are retained, whereas small-amplitude echoes of higher Doppler frequencies are suppressed, the motion of the tissues can be monitored. This will be touched upon again in Chapter 6. An amplitude threshold can be set to allow only the larger echoes to pass through. Tissue Doppler has been proven a clinically useful tool for assessing the state of myocardium.

In conventional pulsed Doppler, only one gate is used to measure blood flow within the sampled window or sampling volume confined by the beam width and the gate duration. If blood flow velocities at multiple points along the ultrasound beam need to be measured, pulsed Doppler flowmeters with multiple gates, e.g., 8 or 16 gates, have been developed. These devices allow the measurements of velocities in real time across the lumen, and thus have been used frequently to determine the blood flow velocity profile in arteries.

References and Further Reading Materials

Evans DH and McDicken WN. *Doppler ultrasound: Physics, instrumentation and signal processing*. Wiley: New York, 2000.

Feigenbaum H. *Echocardiography*. 4th ed. Philadelphia: Lea and Febiger, 1986.

Jensen JA. *Estimation of blood velocities using ultrasound*. Cambridge: Cambridge University Press, 1996.

Mo LYL and Cobbold RSC. Theoretical models of ultrasonic scattering in blood. In Shung KK and Thieme GA (eds.), *Ultrasonic scattering in biological tissues*. Boca Raton, FL: CRC Press, 1993, pp. 125–170.

Nichols WW and O'Rourke MF. *McDonald's blood flow in arteries*. Philadelphia: Lea and Febiger, 1990.

Shung KK, Cloutier G, and Lim CC. The effects of hematocrit, shear rate, and turbulence on ultrasonic Doppler spectrum from blood. *IEEE Trans Biomed Eng* 1992; 39: 462–469.

chapter six

Flow and displacement imaging

Ultrasonic B-mode real-time imaging can be combined with Doppler in a scanner so that the scanner is capable of providing not only anatomical information, but also blood flow data. Both sets of information are displayed simultaneously. A cursor line is typically superimposed on the B-mode image to indicate the direction of the Doppler beam. A fast Fourier transform (FFT) algorithm is used to compute the Doppler spectrum that is displayed in real time. This type of scanner is called duplex scanner. More recently, electronic and computer speed is fast enough to allow blood flow information superimposed on the B-mode image displayed in real time.

6.1 Color Doppler flow imaging

Color Doppler flow imaging systems are duplex scanners capable of displaying both B-mode and Doppler blood flow data simultaneously in real time (Shung et al., 1992; Routh, 1996; Jensen, 1996; Ferrara and DeAngelis, 1997). The Doppler information is encoded in color. Conventionally the color red is assigned to indicate flow toward the transducer, and the color blue is assigned to indicate flow away from the transducer. The magnitude of the velocity is represented by different shades of the color. Typically the lighter the color, the higher the velocity. The color Doppler image is superimposed on the gray-scale B-mode image. A color Doppler image of carotid bifurcation in the neck is shown in Figure 6.1.

The basic concept of the color Doppler is similar to that of the pulsed Doppler instruments that extract the mean Doppler shift frequency from a sample volume defined by the beam width and the gate width. The only exception is that the color Doppler instruments are capable of estimating the mean Doppler shifts of many sample volumes along a scan line in a very short period of time, on the order of 30 to 50 ms. The most straightforward way of achieving this is to compute the FFT from each sample volume and then to calculate the mean frequency from the Fourier spectrum. Unfortunately, current electronic and computer technology cannot yet do that. To be able to do so, fast algorithms have to be developed.

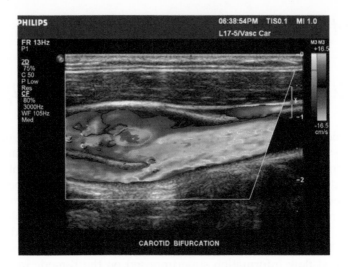

Figure 6.1 Color Doppler image of a carotid artery bifurcation. Blood flow is represented by the color image, whereas the gray-scale B-mode image delineates the arterial anatomy. (Courtesy of Philips Medical Systems.)

An approach was derived from considering the phase of a wave. For a plane wave given below,

$$p(z,t) = p_0 e^{i(2\pi ft - kz)} \tag{6.1}$$

where the phase of the wave $\varphi = 2\pi ft - kz$. The first time derivative of φ divided by 2π yields the frequency:

$$f = \frac{1}{2\pi} \frac{\partial \varphi}{\partial t} \tag{6.2}$$

If the phase of a plane wave can be estimated, the frequency at a certain time may be approximated by the slope of the phase at that time, as shown in Figure 6.2, represented by the following equation:

$$f \approx \frac{1}{2\pi} \frac{\varphi_m - \varphi_{m-1}}{\Delta t} \tag{6.3}$$

where φ_m and φ_{m-1} denote the phases at two different times at $m\Delta t$ and $(m-1)\Delta t$. For a complex function like the plane wave, $p(z,t) = r(z,t) + ji(z,t)$, where

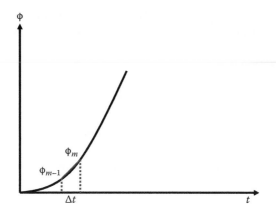

Figure 6.2 The frequency of a wave can be estimated approximately by the slope of the phase at time *t*.

r and *i* represent the real and imaginary parts of the complex number. The phase term is given by

$$\varphi = \tan^{-1} \frac{i(z,t)}{r(z,t)} \tag{6.4}$$

Substituting Equation (6.3) into Equation (6.4), the phase term can be estimated from

$$f = \frac{1}{2\pi\Delta t}\left[\tan^{-1}\frac{i(z,m\Delta t)}{r(z,\,m\Delta t)} - \tan^{-1}\frac{i\big(z,(m-1)\Delta t\big)}{r\big(z,\,(m-1)\Delta t\big)}\right] \tag{6.5}$$

One such algorithm for estimating frequency from the phase of a wave was based upon the well-known Wiener–Khinchine theorem, which shows that the autocorrelation function $H(\tau)$ of a complex function $p(t)$ is the Fourier transform of the power spectrum $P(\omega)$ of $p(t)$ (Kasai et al., 1985). Mathematically, this is given by

$$H(\tau) = \int_{-\infty}^{\infty} p(t)p(t-\tau)\,dt = \int_{-\infty}^{\infty} P(\omega)e^{j\omega\tau}d\omega \tag{6.6}$$

Alternatively, $H(\tau)$ can be written in the form of

$$H(\tau) = |H(\tau)|\,e^{j\varphi(\tau)} = A(\tau)e^{j\varphi(\tau)} \tag{6.7}$$

where the magnitude and phase of $H(\tau)$ are, respectively, an even function and an odd function. The symbol A is used to represent the magnitude of $H(\tau)$ here.

From Equation (6.6),

$$H(0) = \int_{-\infty}^{\infty} P(\omega)d\omega \tag{6.8}$$

$$\dot{H}(0) = j\int_{-\infty}^{\infty} \omega P(\omega)d\omega \tag{6.9}$$

where the dot operation represents the first derivative $= \partial H(\tau)/\partial \tau$. Let $<\omega>$ denote the mean of ω, and from the definition of mean angular frequency and Equations (6.8) and (6.9),

$$<\omega> = \frac{\displaystyle\int_{-\infty}^{\infty} \omega P(\omega)d\omega}{\displaystyle\int_{-\infty}^{\infty} P(\omega)d\omega} = \frac{\dot{H}(0)}{jH(0)} \tag{6.10}$$

This equation can be manipulated to become

$$j<\omega> = \frac{\dot{H}(0)}{H(0)} \tag{6.11}$$

Further, the variance of angular frequency, σ^2, is given by

$$\sigma^2 = <\omega^2> - <\omega>^2 \tag{6.12}$$

The term $<\omega>^2$ can be calculated from Equation (6.10), and $<\omega^2>$ by definition is

$$<\omega^2> = \frac{\displaystyle\int_{-\infty}^{\infty} \omega^2 P(\omega)d\omega}{\displaystyle\int_{-\infty}^{\infty} P(\omega)d\omega} = \frac{-\ddot{H}(0)}{H(0)} \tag{6.13}$$

where the double dot operation denotes the second derivative $= \partial^2 H(\tau)/\partial \tau^2$.

Substituting Equation (6.13) into Equation (6.12),

$$\sigma^2 = \left[\frac{\dot{H}(0)}{H(0)}\right]^2 - \frac{\ddot{H}(0)}{H(0)} \tag{6.14}$$

It can be further shown that for an ultrasonic imaging system transmitting pulses with a pulse repetition frequency T,

$$< \omega > = \frac{\varphi(T)}{T} \tag{6.15}$$

$$\sigma^2 = \frac{1}{T^2} \left[1 - \frac{|H(T)|}{H(0)} \right] \tag{6.16}$$

These are all simple arithmetic operations that require little time for computation if the autocorrelation function $H(T)$ can be estimated.

Equations (6.15) and (6.16) can be found by considering the fact that for an even function, the first derivative of the function at the origin $= 0$, and for an odd function, the function $= 0$ at the origin, i.e.,

$$\dot{A}(0) = \frac{\partial |H(\tau)|}{\partial \tau}\bigg|_{\tau=0} = 0 \quad and \quad \varphi(0) = 0 \tag{6.17}$$

Therefore,

$$\dot{H}(0) = \dot{A}(0)e^{j\varphi(0)} + jA(0)e^{j\varphi(0)}\dot{\varphi}(0) = jA(0)\dot{\varphi}(0) \tag{6.18}$$

From Equations (6.11) and (6.18),

$$< \omega > = \dot{\varphi}(0) \approx \frac{\varphi(T) - \varphi(0)}{T} = \frac{\varphi(T)}{T}$$

which is Equation (6.15). This expression says that the mean frequency of a spectrum is equal to the slope of the phase of the autocorrelation function at the origin that can be approximated by the difference in phase at the origin and at one pulse repetition period T, assuming that the autocorrelation function is sampled at internals of T. Similarly, it can be shown from differentiating $H(\tau)$ twice that

$$\ddot{H}(0) = \ddot{A}(0) - [\dot{\varphi}(0)]^2 A(0) \tag{6.19}$$

Here $A(\tau)$ can be expanded into a Taylor series, ignoring third-order and higher terms and assuming that τ is small,

$$A(\tau) \approx A(0) + \frac{\tau^2}{2}\ddot{A}(0) \tag{6.20}$$

Rearranging Equation (6.19),

$$\ddot{A}(0) = \frac{2}{\tau^2}[A(\tau) - A(0)] \tag{6.21}$$

$\dot{H}(0)$ can be found by substituting Equation (6.21) into Equation (6.19). Substituting $\dot{H}(0)$, $\ddot{H}(0)$, and $H(0)$ into Equation (6.14), Equation (6.16) is obtained.

$$\sigma^2 \approx \frac{2}{\tau^2}\left[1 - \frac{A(\tau)}{A(0)}\right] \approx \frac{2}{T^2}\left[1 - \frac{|H(T)|}{H(0)}\right]$$

This expression indicates that the variance of the frequency can be estimated from the magnitude of the autocorrelation function at the origin and at T.

Figure 6.3 shows a version of the autocorrelation method that was implemented in a commercial scanner a few years ago. Given a real-time function $f(t)$, its quadrature component $g(t)$ can be found by shifting the time function by 90°. A complex function $z(t) = f(t) + jg(t)$ can be obtained. The complex multiplier performs the operation

$$[f(t) + jg(t)] \cdot [f(t - T) - jg(t - T)]$$

The autocorrelation function is obtained by integrating the output of the complex multiplier over a period of time, say nT, where n represents the successive pulses transmitted by a scanner to acquire the autocorrelation function.

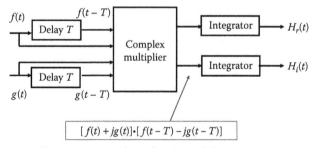

Compute autocorrelation function and then average

Figure 6.3 A hardwired autocorrelator for estimating the autocorrelation function $H(T)$ from a time signal $f(t)$.

The three unknowns in Equations (6.15) and (6.16) are readily attainable from the following expressions:

$$|H(T)| = \sqrt{H_r^{2}(T) + H_i^{2}(T)} \quad and \quad \varphi(T) = \tan^{-1}\frac{H_i(T)}{H_r(T)}$$

where H_r and H_i are the real and imaginary parts of H.

It should be noted that $H(T)$ is a function of time or is time dependent. The accuracy of the estimated $H(T)$ is ultimately determined by the time duration in which the estimation is performed. The longer the time duration, the better the accuracy. This requirement must be comprised in real-time ultrasonic imaging. In the earliest color Doppler scanners, there were 50 scan lines with a frame rate of 15 per second. The dwelling time of the ultrasound beam at any one direction is

$$t_d = \frac{1}{50 \cdot 15} = 1.33\,ms$$

If the depth of view is 10 cm, the time needed for a pulse to make a round-trip or time of flight is 0.13 ms assuming an ultrasound speed of 1540 m/s. This means that 1.33/0.13 = 10 ultrasound pulses can be transmitted in this time span, and that the autocorrelation function is computed and averaged after 10 pulse transmissions. The autocorrelator needs to compute the autocorrelation function for each pixel along a scan line, as illustrated in Figure 6.4, where the thin curve and the thick curve

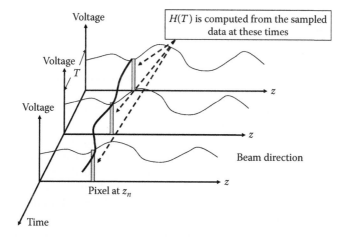

Figure 6.4 The autocorrelation function from which the mean and the variance of the Doppler-shifted frequency are estimated is computed for each pixel along a scan line in a color Doppler flow mapping system.

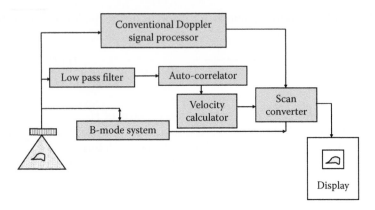

Figure 6.5 Block diagram of a color Doppler flow mapping system.

represent, respectively, the pulse-echo waveform after each pulse transmission and the time variation of the echo at a certain pixel for which the autocorrelation function is computed.

In a color Doppler system, the signal received by a probe is divided into three paths, one for constructing the gray-scale B-mode image, one for calculating the flow information from Doppler data using a hardwired autocorrelator, and one for conventional Doppler measurements. This is delineated in Figure 6.5. Eight or more shades are used in these systems to depict the magnitude of the velocity. The higher the velocity, the lighter the shade. Since the basic principle of Doppler flow mapping is similar to that of pulsed Doppler, the maximal Doppler frequency that can be detected without aliasing is half of the pulse repetition frequency. Therefore, a higher pulse repetition frequency is favored for avoiding aliasing and increasing the accuracy of the autocorrelation. However, limited by the frame rate and field of view, the pulse repetition frequency in most color Doppler systems is between 8 and 16 KHz, frequently resulting in aliasing with color Doppler in cardiac imaging. To overcome these problems, the image size may be reduced, or M-mode color Doppler where the beam is fixed in one direction may be used.

In the heart, the myocardium is in motion during a cardiac cycle, and tissue color Doppler images of this motion can also be acquired with the color Doppler methods previously described. The difference lies in that myocardial motion is slower than blood flow and myocardial echoes are stronger than blood. The spurious Doppler signals from blood in this case can be eliminated by thresholding the echoes as illustrated in Figure 6.6. A tissue Doppler image of the heart where the color indicates the velocity of myocardial motion is shown in Figure 6.7.

Many clinical applications have been found for color Doppler flow imaging, including diagnosing tiny shunts in the heart wall and valvular

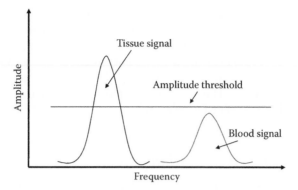

Figure 6.6 Tissue Doppler can be achieved by thresholding the Doppler signals so as to suppress the Doppler signal from blood and retain only the Doppler signals from tissues.

regurgitation and stenosis. It considerably reduces the examination time in many diseases associated with flow disturbance. Problematic regions can be quickly identified first from the flow mapping. More quantitative conventional Doppler measurements are then made on these areas.

Although color Doppler has now been widely used in a variety of medical disciplines, it has several shortcomings. (1) Flow perpendicular to the beam cannot be reliably detected. (2) Higher blood flow velocity results in aliasing. (3) Its spatial resolution is poorer than B-mode gray-scale imaging. (4) The mean velocity estimated is the average velocity

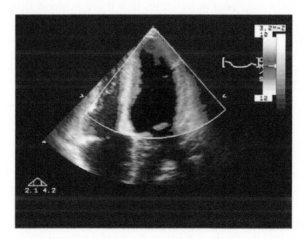

Figure 6.7 Tissue Doppler image of myocardial motion. Colored areas indicate velocity of myocardium motion in the heart walls, and anechoic regions indicate intracardiac blood pool. (Courtesy of Philips Medical Systems.)

within a pixel or voxel. (5) Since the color Doppler image is overlaid over the gray-scale B-mode, the overlay process is determined arbitrarily by thresholding, which may result in vessel-wall overwrite obscuring the slow blood flow signal near the wall. (6) Large echoes due to slow-moving tissues can cause the "color flash artifact" because they overlap echoes from flowing blood. (7) The frame rate is reduced because separate firing is needed to obtain a color Doppler image.

6.2 Color Doppler power imaging

Another way of displaying the color Doppler information, i.e., power mode or energy mode imaging, has been introduced to minimize some of the color Doppler problems (Rubin et al., 1994; Zagzebski, 1996). Instead of the mean Doppler shift, the power contained in the Doppler signal is displayed in this approach. There are several advantages to doing so. (1) A threshold can be set to minimize the effect of noise. (2) The data can be averaged to achieve a better signal-to-noise ratio. (3) The images are less dependent upon the Doppler angle. Finally, (4) aliasing is no longer a problem since only the power is detected. Because of these advantages, signals from blood flowing in much smaller vessels may be detected. The images so produced have an appearance similar to that of x-ray angiography preferred by radiologists. The disadvantages of this approach are that (1) it is more susceptible to motion artifacts due to frame averaging and (2) the image contains no information on flow velocity and direction. A color power Doppler image of a carotid artery bifurcation is shown in Figure 6.8. The orange region indicates that there is blood flow. The gray-scale B-mode image delineates blood vessel wall and surrounding tissues.

Power Doppler imaging is in fact easier to implement than conventional color Doppler because Doppler power is readily available in conventional color Doppler systems. $H(0)$ in Equation (6.11), which is needed to calculate the mean Doppler frequency, is the power contained in the Doppler spectrum. This becomes apparent when setting $\tau = 0$ in Equation (6.6), i.e.,

$$H(\tau = 0) = \int\limits_{-\infty}^{\infty} p^2(t)dt = \int_{-\infty}^{\infty} P(\omega)d\omega$$

6.3 Time domain flow estimation

Blood flow velocity has been estimated directly from B-mode images, termed speckle tracking, or from radio frequency (RF) echoes. These alternatives accomplish flow blood measurements in the time domain.

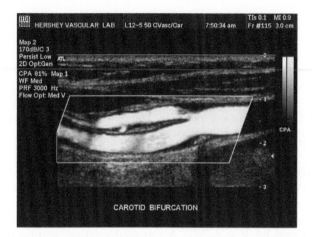

Figure 6.8 Color power Doppler image of carotid artery acquired with a 12 MHz linear array. The color in this case represents the power contained in the Doppler signal rather than the mean Doppler-shifted frequency. The brightness of the color is proportional to the Doppler power and has nothing to do with the magnitude of velocity. The presence of a color in a pixel merely means that a flow signal is detected in that pixel. (Courtesy of Philips ATL.)

Both frame-to-frame tracking of movement of speckles generated by blood from B-mode images and direct correlation of RF echoes from blood show great promise.

Suppose that an ultrasonic beam emanating from a transducer is parallel to blood flowing in a vessel and a signal $e(t)$ is received by the transducer from blood, as shown in Figure 6.9. For frame-to-frame speckle

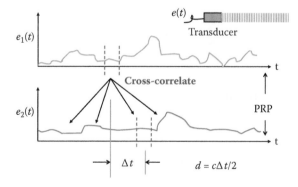

Figure 6.9 Cross-correlation can be used to estimate blood flow in the time domain: $V = d/T = cDt/(2T)$ where d is the distance that the blood has moved In one PRP - T.

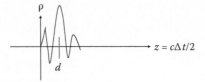

Figure 6.10 Cross-correlation coefficient computed as a function of separation distance of two volumes being correlated.

tracking, $e(t)$ denotes video signal. If RF signals are used, then $e(t)$ denotes RF signal. Waveforms $e_1(t)$ and $e_2(t)$ are received at times t_1 and t_2, which are separated by the pulse repetition period (PRP). If the distance, d, that the blood has moved within one PRP can be measured, the velocity, V, would be given by $V = d/PRP$. A cross-correlation approach has been developed to estimate the distance d (Trahey et al., 1987; Jensen, 1996). A segment of the waveform or the windowed waveform in a pixel, bordered by the dashed lines of $e_1(t)$ in Figure 6.9, is cross-correlated with all segments of similar width of waveform $e_2(t)$ by computing the one-dimensional normalized cross-correlation coefficient, ρ. A match is found when ρ is maximal, shown in Figure 6.10. If the windowed waveforms are represented by N digitized signals $E_1 = \{e_1(0), e_1(1), ..., e_1(i), ..., e_1(N-1)\}$ and $E_2 = \{e_2(0), e_2(1), ..., e_2(i), ..., e_2(N-1)\}$, the normalized coefficient ρ can be computed from the following expression, as E_1 is correlated with different E_2 segments from waveform $e_2(t)$ by shifting the window from one end of the waveform to the other.

$$\rho = \frac{\sum_{i=0}^{N-1} [e_1(i) - \bar{e}_1][e_2(i) - \bar{e}_2]}{\sqrt{\sum_{i=0}^{N-1} [e_1(i) - \bar{e}_1]^2 \sum_{i=0}^{N-1} [e_2(i) - \bar{e}_2]^2}} \tag{6.22}$$

where $\bar{e}_1$ and $\bar{e}_2$ are the mean values of e_1 and e_2. If maximal ρ occurs when the windowed waveform of $e_2(t)$ is shifted Δt from the windowed segment of $e_1(t)$, it may be assumed that the volume of blood responsible for the windowed $e_1(t)$ has moved a distance $d = c\Delta t/2$, where c is ultrasound velocity. Consequently, blood flow velocity can be estimated from

$$V = \frac{c\Delta t}{2T} \tag{6.23}$$

where T is the pulse repetition period (PRP). If the ultrasound beam makes an angle of θ relative to the flow direction, Equation (6.23) should be modified to include the effect of the angle.

$$V = \frac{c\Delta t}{2T\cos\theta} \tag{6.24}$$

Time domain methods differ from Doppler methods in that they track displacements. These methods can still be used when there is no motion, but Doppler cannot. They have several advantages over Doppler methods. (1) Time domain methods are more immune to noise. This means that they can be used in a noisier environment and need less averaging, yielding a higher frame rate. (2) There is no aliasing problem. The search will yield no results if the pulse repetition frequency is not sufficiently high. (3) The spatial resolution attainable with these methods is higher than that with Doppler methods because short pulses are used. (4) 2D flow information can be obtained by matching 2D blocks by the computing 2D correlation coefficient.

The frame-to-frame speckle tracking is more desirable in that the flow information can be directly obtained from the B-mode images that are acquired by the scanner without the need for additional hardware, although it yields poorer spatial resolution than RF correlation. Its drawbacks are that the signal level from blood in the frequency range of 3 to 10 MHz is too weak to obtain a reliable estimation, and the frame rate of 30 per second is too low to estimate arterial blood flow velocity. The former problem is becoming less of an issue because the performance of recent scanners has been improved, and it may be overcome by injecting a contrast agent, whereas a high frame scanner has to be used to solve the latter problem. Several echocardiographic scanners now are capable of providing a frame rate as high as 200 frames/s with a smaller field of view.

6.4 Elasticity imaging

Ultrasound has been widely used to differentiate cysts from solid tumors in tumor imaging because liquid-containing cysts are typically echo poor. However, certain solid tumors that are harder than surrounding tissues are oftentimes missed by ultrasound because their echogenicity is similar to that of surrounding tissues. These tumors or harder tissues are identifiable if their elastic properties can be imaged. Several ultrasound approaches have been developed to image tissue elasticity, which may be classified into two categories: static and dynamic (Ophir et al., 1991; Lerner et al., 1990; Fatemi and Greenleaf, 1998; Nightingale et al., 2002; Bercoff et al., 2004).

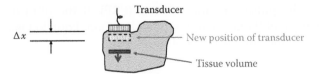

Figure 6.11 A plate pressed against a body of tissue induces displacement of a volume of tissue in the direction of the force.

6.4.1 Elastography

In one static approach dubbed elastography (Ophir et al., 1991), a flat plate that may be the ultrasonic probe itself is used to compress the tissue by a distance Δz; the displacement of the tissue is estimated via cross-correlation from the returned RF echoes, as previously discussed, illustrated in Figure 6.11. Under idealistic conditions, assuming a 1D case, i.e., the compression is transmitted only in the z-direction, the stress and strain can be estimated from the force applied and area of the plate or transducer and Δz, respectively. The Young's modulus of the tissue is then given by the ratio of the longitudinal stress to the longitudinal strain. This idea can be illustrated by the following simple example, illustrated in Figure 6.12(a), where media I and II are perfectly compressible and incompressible. When a stress κ is applied, all points in medium I will be displaced by Δz, whereas in medium II, the displacement

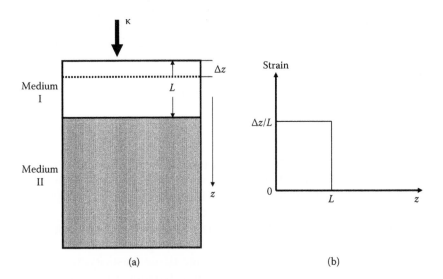

Figure 6.12 (a) A stress applied to medium I produces a displacement in medium I. (b) Strain in medium I and II is plotted as a function of depth.

Multifocal breast cancer *in vivo*

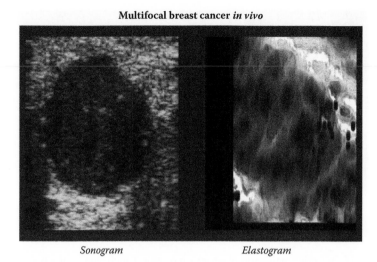

Sonogram   *Elastogram*

Figure 6.13 A comparison of elastogram and B-mode image of a multiple-foci breast lesion. (Courtesy of Dr. Jonathan Ophir at University of Texas Medical School at Houston.)

will be 0. This is plotted in Figure 6.12(b), where the strain in medium I is given by $-(\Delta z)/L$ and the Young's modulus $-(L\kappa)/\Delta z$.

This approach has been the focus of attention for a number of years in breast and prostate imaging. An example is shown in Figure 6.13, where the elastogram and B-mode image of a multiple-foci breast lesion are compared. Although elastography may be capable of imaging the elastic property of tissues, which cannot be achieved with standard B-mode sonography, it suffers from problems of the same nature as B-mode sonography. The stress propagating into a tissue will be attenuated by tissues, spread into other directions from the primary incident direction, and interact with a boundary between two media of different elastic properties. The effect of boundary on an elastogram can sometimes be distracting. In addition, its spatial resolution is in general poorer than B-mode ultrasound. This approach has been offered by several manufacturers as an option. For instance, Siemens has adopted this approach in its scanner called eSie Touch. Figure 6.14 shows a B-mode image (left) and an elastogram (right) of a biopsy-proven breast carcinoma. The red color in the elastogram indicates harder tissue.

6.4.2 Sonoelasticity imaging

Sonoelasticity imaging (Lerner et al., 1990) is a dynamic approach in which a motion monitoring device, e.g., a color Doppler flow mapping system,

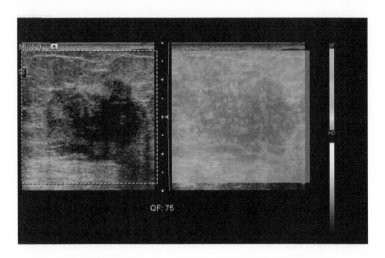

Figure 6.14 B-mode image and elastogram or eSie Touch image of a breast lesion obtained by a Siemens scanner. Red indicates harder tissue in this large breast lesion. (Courtesy of Siemens Medical Systems.)

is used to measure the motion of tissues produced by the vibration of a source inserted into one of the cavities of the body or placed externally, as illustrated in Figure 6.15. The source typically vibrates at a frequency of a few hundred Hz to a few kHz, so that a conventional Doppler device can be used to monitor the motion with little modification. This approach has been used to assess prostate cancer with an intrarectal vibrating source. Sonoelasticity imaging suffers from problems similar to those mentioned previously. The vibration produced by the source is nonuniform and is attenuated by tissues. The energy of the ultrasound generated by the scanner to probe the vibration is also affected by attenuation.

6.5 Acoustic radiation force imaging (ARFI)

As was discussed in Chapter 2, a force is generated by a wave as it propagates into a medium. The force pushes the medium forward, producing a displacement of the medium. Nightingale et al. (2002) pioneered a method that utilizes the acoustic radiation force produced by a propagating ultrasonic beam to image elastic properties of a tissue. In their approach a commercial Siemens 7.2 MHz linear array was modified to fire a pushing beam

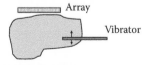

Figure 6.15 Sonoelasticity imaging of motion of tissues induced by a vibrator.

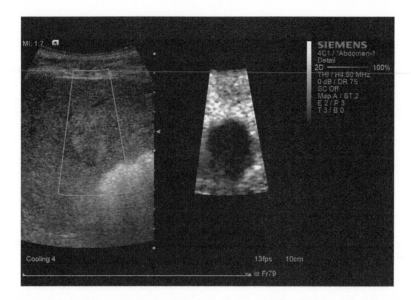

Figure 6.16 B-mode image and ARFI or Virtual Touch image of a liver lesion obtained by a Siemens scanner. (Courtesy of Siemens Medical Systems.)

with a pulse duration of a fraction of a ms and an imaging beam with a pulse duration of a fraction of a μs and a PRF of a few kHz consecutively. Ultrasonic images were acquired at a rate of approximately 3 frames/s. A commercial version at a much higher frame rate (13 frames/s) is now available on Siemens scanners, called Virtual Touch. Figure 6.16 shows a Virtual Touch image (right) of a lesion in liver produced by a Siemens scanner. The image on the left is a B-mode image. In this case, the contrast of the ARFI image is much better than that of the B-mode image. ARFI is now available on other commercial scanners as well.

6.6 Vibro-acoustography

The term *vibro-acoustography* (VA) was coined by Fatemi and Greenleaf (1998). In this approach two ultrasonic beams are sent to a region of interest located at the intersection of two beams, as shown in Figure 6.17. These two beams interfere, producing a beat frequency that is the difference of the incident frequencies. The amplitude of the emitted signal at the beat frequency is related to the elastic properties of the medium where the two beams intersect. It can be detected by a hydrophone. An image is formed if the transducer assembly is scanned and its spatial position encoded like a C-scan system. Figure 6.18(a) shows a prone cranial caudal x-ray mammogram image of the left breast with a 2 cm diameter calcified fibroadenoma. Figure 6.18(b) shows the VA image at 40 kHz and in 2.5 cm depth

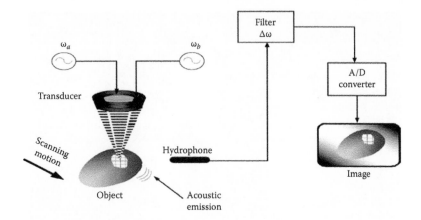

Figure 6.17 Schematic diagram of vibro-acoustography. (Courtesy of Dr. Mostafa Fatemi of Mayo Clinic.)

from the skin, whereas (c) shows the VA image at 50 KHz and in 3 cm depth. The VA images clearly show the lesion and other structures within the breast with high contrast and no speckle.

6.7 Supersonic shear wave imaging (SSWI)

Although shear wave propagation in biological tissues is heavily attenuated, as was discussed in Chapter 2, and may be ignored for practical purposes, more recently it has been shown that it is possible to propagate shear wave in tissues (Bercoff et al., 2004). In fact, the local propagation speed of the shear wave in a tissue, typically a few meters per second, is related to its elastic properties given by Equation (2.14). Low-frequency shear wave is generated in tissues in SSWI with the same kind of linear arrays used in

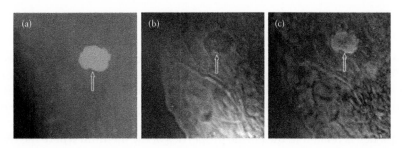

Figure 6.18 (a) Prone cranial caudal x-ray mammogram image of the left breast. This image shows a 2 cm diameter calcified fibroadenoma. (b) VA image at 40 kHz and in 2.5 cm depth from the skin. (c) VA image at 50 KHz and in 3 cm depth. The VA images show the lesion and other structures within the breast with high contrast and no speckle. (Courtesy of Dr. Mostafa Fatemi of Mayo Clinic.)

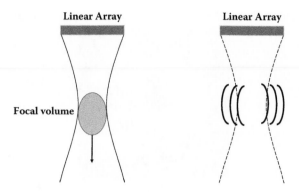

Figure 6.19 Two phases of supersonic shear wave imaging: (a) pushing and (b) imaging.

B-mode imaging, as illustrated in Figure 6.19. A highly focused pushing beam generates a shear wave propagating perpendicularly to the incident beam. The shear wave is imaged with a high frame rate scanner (up to 6000 frames/s) using the same array, which generates plane wave incidence achieved by properly applying delays in beamforming to monitor and estimate the local tissue longitudinal displacement induced by the acoustic radiation force generated by the shear wave. Tissue displacement estimation is carried out by cross-correlating the acquired echo signal to the reference echo data set collected prior to pushing. Bercoff et al. (2004) further demonstrated that by sending consecutive ultrasonic pulses, it is possible to generate supersonic plane shear waves propagating perpendicularly to the incident beam, much like the sonic boom phenomenon, because ultrasonic longitudinal propagation speed is much faster than shear wave speed. This is delineated in Figure 6.20(a) and (b), which is an

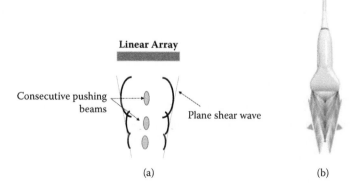

Figure 6.20 (a) Consecutive firing of pushing beams produces two plane shear waves. (b) Animation. (Courtesy of Supersonic Imagine.)

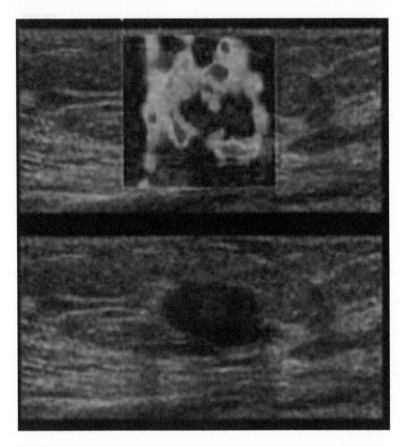

Figure 6.21 Upper: Supersonic shear wave image. Lower: B-mode image of a breast lesion. (Courtesy of Supersonic Imagine.)

animation. Figure 6.21 shows a supersonic shear wave image (upper) of a breast ductal carcinoma obtained *in vivo*, where different color indicates different elasticity, and a B-mode image of the same lesion (lower).

6.8 B-Flow imaging

B-mode blood flow (B-flow) imaging is a new method that improves the resolution, frame rate, and dynamic range of B-mode to simultaneously image both blood flow and tissue (Chiao et al., 2000). It combines the coded excitation imaging previously described in Chapter 5 with a scheme to equalize tissue signals, which is necessitated by the fact that tissue echoes are often much stronger than those from blood. The gray scale of an echo is adjusted by correlating the echo waveforms temporally. The correlation function measures the similarity of two echo waveforms

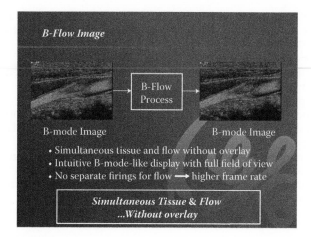

Figure 6.22 A comparison of B-mode and B-flow images obtained from a carotid artery. (Courtesy of GE Medical Systems.)

and is determined by blood echogenicity, blood flow velocity, and beam width. A filter is designed to suppress large and slow- or nonmoving echoes. The result is that the image of blood is enhanced so as to allow the better visualization of blood flow, especially close to the vessel wall. A comparison of the B-mode and B-flow images of a carotid artery is shown in Figure 6.22. It is evident that blood flow is better visualized by B-flow imaging. The vessel lumen where blood flows in the B-mode image is basically anechoic.

References and Further Reading Materials

Bercoff J, Tanter M, and Fink M. Supersonic shear imaging: A new technique for soft tissue elasticity mapping. *IEEE Trans Ultrasonics Ferroelect Freq Cont* 2004; 51: 396–409.

Chiao RY, Mo LY, Hall AL, Miller SC, and Thomenius K. B-mode blood flow imaging. In Schneider SC, Levy M, and McAvoy BR (eds.), *Proceedings of 2000 IEEE Ultrasonics Symposium*, New York, 2000, pp. 1469–1472.

Ferrara K and DeAngelis G. Color Doppler mapping. *Ultrasound Med Biol* 1997; 23: 321–345.

Fatemi H and Greenleaf JM. Ultrasound-stimulated vibro-acoustic spectrography. *Science* 1998; 280: 82–85.

Jensen JA. *Estimation of blood velocities using ultrasound.* Cambridge: Cambridge Press, 1996.

Kasai C, Namekawa K, Koyano A, and Omoto R. Real-time two-dimensional blood flow imaging using an autocorrelation technique. *IEEE Trans Sonics Ultrasonics* 1985; 32: 458–463.

Lerner RM, Huang SR, and Parker K. Sonoelasticity images derived from ultrasound signals in mechanically vibrated tissues. *Ultrasound Med Biol* 1990; 16: 231–239.

Nightingale KR, Soo MS, Nightingale RW, and Trahey GE. Acoustic radiation force impulse imaging: *In vivo* demonstration of clinical feasibility. *Ultrasound Med Biol* 2002; 28: 227–235.

Ophir J, Cespedes I, Ponnekanti H, Yazdi Y, and Li X. Elastography: A quantitative method for imaging the elasticity of biological tissues. *Ultrasonic Imaging* 1991; 13: 111–134.

Routh H. Doppler ultrasound. *Engr Med Biol Mag* 1996; 15:31–40.

Rubin M, Bude RO, Carson PL, Bree RL, and Adler RS. Power Doppler US: A potentially useful alternative to mean frequency-based color Doppler US. *Radiology* 1994; 190: 853–856.

Shung KK, Smith MB, and Tsui B. *Principles of medical imaging*. San Diego: Academic Press, 1992.

Trahey GE, Allison JW, and von Ramm OT. Angle independent ultrasonic detection of blood flow. *IEEE Trans Biomed Eng* 1987; 34: 965–967.

Zagzebski JA. *Essentials of ultrasound physics*. St. Louis, MO: Mosby, 1996.

chapter seven

Contrast media and harmonic imaging

Contrast media have been used very extensively in radiology, cardiology, and other medical disciplines to enhance certain anatomical structures in an image. For instance, iodinated compounds can be injected into the coronary artery to better visualize the coronary vasculature in the heart, either intravenously or intra-arterially. Similarly, ultrasonic contrast agents have been successfully developed (Goldberg et al., 1994; de Jong, 1996; Chang and Shung, 1998; Wilson and Burns, 2010), and many applications, including imaging of cardiac chambers, tumor vasculature, and blood flow in various organs, including the kidney and liver, have been found. Their ultimate application may well be in quantitating perfusion that is blood supply to a certain region of the organ, which is a yet unattainable goal by many imaging modalities. Encapsulated ultrasonic gaseous contrast agents where drug may be loaded have been studied for drug delivery (Ferrara et al., 2007). More recently, ultrasonic contrast agents conjugated with targeting ligands have been developed for molecular imaging (Gessner and Dayton, 2010).

7.1 Contrast agents

The primary requirements of an ultrasonic contrast agent are that it is (1) nontoxic, (2) more echogenic than tissues, (3) capable of traversing pulmonary circulation, (4) stable, and (5) uniform in size. Requirement 3 is dictated by the need for intravenous injection that would minimize the risk of intra-arterial injection. To allow the applications of these agents to imaging left cardiac structures and other parts of the body, e.g., the liver and kidney via intravenous injection, they must be smaller than a few microns and stable so that they can traverse the pulmonary circulation. They need to persist at least for a duration of longer than a few tens of seconds. To satisfy the second requirement, a majority of these agents utilize microscopic air bubbles, which are extremely strong ultrasound scatterers because of the acoustic impedance mismatch.

7.1.1 Gaseous agents

Echogenic gaseous bubbles are produced by chemical action or mechanical agitation. Rigorous stirring of a saline solution has been shown to produce air bubbles with a wide distribution of sizes. These bubbles, however, typically would have a very short lifetime, in the order of a few seconds. Insonication of a saline solution is capable of achieving the same result. A microscopic photograph of bubbles generated this way is shown in Figure 7.1. Surface agents may be added to stabilize these bubbles. Air bubbles have not only the advantage of an acoustic impedance mismatch, giving rise to stronger scattering, but also a favorable characteristic in that they resonate when insonified by an ultrasonic wave. The echoes from the bubbles can be further enhanced if the incident wave is tuned to the resonant frequency of the bubbles (Leighton, 1994). The resonant frequency for a free air bubble, a bubble without a shell, f_r, is related to the radius of the bubble, a, by

$$f_r = \frac{1}{2\pi a} \sqrt{\frac{3\gamma P_0}{\rho_w}} \tag{7.1}$$

where γ is the ratio of the specific heats at constant pressure and constant volume of gas and equals 1.4 for air, P_0 is the hydrostatic ambient pressure and equals $1.013 \cdot 10^5$ pascal or $1.013 \cdot 10^6$ dynes/cm^2 at 1 atm, and

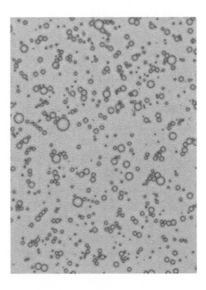

Figure 7.1 A photo of air bubbles generated by agitating saline solution. (Courtesy of Dr. Diane Dalecki, University of Rochester.)

ρ_w is the density of the surrounding medium, e.g., water. The scattering cross section at 2 MHz and resonant frequency of an air bubble of 3 μm radius can be easily calculated from Equations (2.38) and (7.1), assuming that the compressibility and density of air are, respectively, $6.9 \cdot 10^{-7}$ cm^2/dyne and $1.3 \cdot 10^{-3}$ g/cm^3. Here it is assumed that the compressibility term dominates so that the density term can be neglected. Also, G_e in the present case is $\gg G$.

$$\sigma_s = \frac{4}{9}\pi\left(\frac{2\pi}{770\cdot 10^{-4}}\right)^4 (3\cdot 10^{-4})^6\left(\frac{6.9\cdot 10^{-7}}{4.6\cdot 10^{-11}}\right)^2$$

$$= 1.04\cdot 10^{-5}\ \text{cm}^2$$

This is much greater than the scattering cross section of a red cell at 2 MHz. The resonant frequency for an air bubble of 3 μm radius is

$$f_r = \frac{1}{2\pi\cdot 3\cdot 10^{-4}}\sqrt{\frac{3\cdot(1.4)\cdot(1.013\cdot 10^6)}{1.0}}$$

$$= 1.1\times 10^6\ \text{Hz or 1.1 MHz}$$

If the bubble radius is decreased to 1.7 μm so as to resonate at 2 MHz, the scattering strength from a bubble may be further increased. The resonant frequency of a bubble as a function of radius is shown in Figure 7.2. Under the conditions that the bubble size is much smaller than the

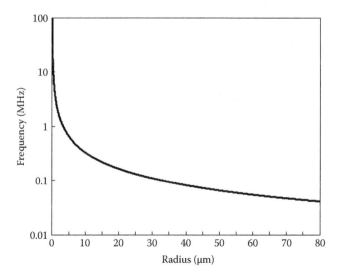

Figure 7.2 Calculated resonance frequency versus radius of a free air bubble.

wavelength, the bubble wall displacement is much smaller than its radius, and the surrounding fluid is incompressible, the scattering cross section of a bubble is given by (Medwin, 1977)

$$\sigma_s = \frac{4\pi a^2}{(f_r^2/f^2 - 1)^2 + \chi^2} \tag{7.2}$$

where a is the radius of the bubble, f_r is the resonant frequency, f is the frequency of the incident wave, and χ is the damping constant consisting of three terms: damping due to reradiation of the ultrasound energy, thermal conductivity (energy loss due to thermal diffusion), and shear viscosity of the surrounding medium (energy loss due to friction).

Equation (7.1) can be rewritten as

$$f_r = \frac{1}{2\pi}\sqrt{\frac{S_a}{m}} \tag{7.3}$$

where S_a is the adiabatic stiffness of the bubble–fluid system defined as (change in force/change in displacement) $= 12\pi\gamma P_0 a$, and m is the effective mass or radiation mass of the system $= 4\pi a^3 \rho_w$. Here an adiabatic equation of state is assumed. However, for bubbles of small radii, surface tension becomes a significant additional restoring force and needs to be considered. Bubble oscillation in this case is better approximated by an isothermal process. Taking these factors into account, P_0 in Equation (7.1) is replaced by the average interior pressure, including surface tension, ςP_0, and γ by the effective ratio of specific heats in the presence of thermal conductivity, $b\gamma$, where b and ς are given by

$$b = (1+B^2)^{-1}\left[1+\frac{3(\gamma-1)}{\xi}\left(\frac{\sinh\xi - \sin\xi}{\cosh\xi - \cos\xi}\right)\right]^{-1} \tag{7.4}$$

$$\varsigma = 1 + \frac{2\delta}{P_0 a}\left(1 - \frac{1}{3\gamma b}\right) \tag{7.5}$$

In Equations (7.4) and (7.5), δ is surface tension $= 75$ dyne/cm for an air bubble,

$$B = 3(\gamma+1)\frac{\xi(\sinh\xi + \sin\xi) - 2(\cosh\xi - \cos\xi)}{\xi^2(\cosh\xi - \cos\xi) + 3(\gamma-1)\xi(\sinh\xi - \sin\xi)} \tag{7.6}$$

$$\xi = a(2\omega\rho_g C_{pg}/K_g)^{1/2} \tag{7.7}$$

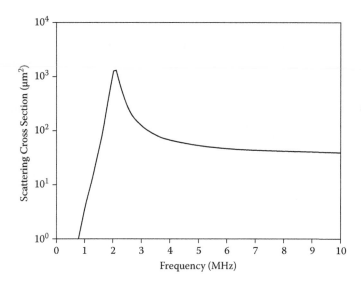

Figure 7.3 Calculated scattering cross section for a free bubble of 1.7 μm radius.

where K_g is the thermal conductivity of air = $5.6 \cdot 10^{-5}$ cal/cm-s-°C, ρ_g is the density of air at sea level = $1.3 \cdot 10^{-3}$ g/cm³, C_{pg} is the specific heat at constant pressure for air = 0.24 cal/g, and ω = angular frequency. Including these parameters, Equation (7.1) should be modified to

$$f_r = \frac{1}{2\pi a} \sqrt{\frac{3b\gamma\varsigma P_0}{\rho_w}}$$

(7.8)

The scattering cross section for a bubble of 1.7 μm radius calculated using Equations (7.2) and (7.8) is shown in Figure 7.3. A scattering peak occurs at approximately 2 MHz, the resonant frequency of the bubble.

For a beam of ultrasound propagating in a bubbly medium, attenuation will be caused, as previously described scattering and absorption. However, in this case scattering is more dominant than absorption. For a suspension of bubbles of low concentration where bubble size is smaller than the wavelength, the pressure attenuation coefficient is given by

$$\alpha = \frac{n\sigma_s}{2}$$

where n is the bubble concentration or number of bubbles per unit volume.

7.1.2 Encapsulated gaseous agents

Free air bubbles have a very short lifetime, which is not suitable for human applications. This problem can be overcome by encapsulating air or gas with a shell. A number of commercial products have been developed. The most well known are Albunex and Optison produced by GE Amersham, Definity produced by Lantheus Medical Imaging, and Sonovue produced by Bracco. Optison is an improved version of Albunex, which uses the plasma protein albumin as the shell material. Albunex contains air, whereas Optison contains a large molecule gas, perfluoropropane, which minimizes diffusion of the gas out of the shell, yielding a much longer bubble lifetime produced by insonicating a solution that contains human serum albumin and other ingredients. An electron micrograph of Optison microspheres is shown in Figure 7.4.

The effect of a shell on the resonant behavior may be taken into consideration by assuming that the shell causes an additional restoring force to the bubble system, which tends to increase the resonant frequency and decrease the scattering cross section (de Jong, 1996). The contribution of the shell to the bubble stiffness is given by

$$S_{shell} = 8\pi \frac{El_t}{1 - \upsilon_p} = 8\pi S_p \tag{7.9}$$

where S_{shell} is the shell stiffness, E is Young's modulus, l_t is wall thickness, υ_p is Poisson's ratio of the shell material, and $S_p = El_t/(1 - \upsilon_p)$, the shell stiffness parameter defined as (change in force/change in displacement) in dynes/cm. The resonant frequency of a bubble with a

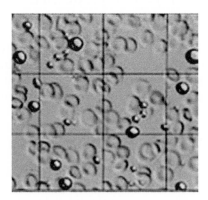

Figure 7.4 An electron micrograph of Optison. (Courtesy of GE Amersham.)

shell can be obtained from Equation (7.3) by including an additional stiffness term:

$$f_r = \frac{1}{2\pi} \sqrt{\frac{b\varsigma S_a + S_{shell}}{m}} \qquad\qquad (7.10)$$

The parameters given in Equation (7.10) are difficult to estimate. It may be done by fitting experimental data to theoretical models. To better fit the experimental data to theory, an additional damping term, which accounted for internal friction or viscosity within the shell, was introduced by de Jong (1996). The optimal value for the shell stiffness of the Albunex microspheres was estimated to be $8 \cdot 10^3$ dynes/cm.

7.1.3 Dilute distribution of bubbles of varying size

It is extremely difficult, if not impossible, to produce bubbles of a very narrow range of size distribution. The sonicated solution typically has a larger size distribution than the commercially produced agents. Albunex has a mean diameter of 3–5 µm, with a large portion of the bubbles with a radius smaller than 10 µm. Figure 7.5 shows the size distribution of Albunex and Optison (FS069). When the volume concentration of the

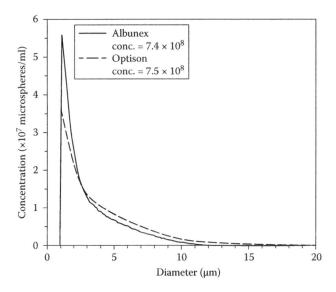

Figure 7.5 Size distributions of two commercial contrast agents, Albunex and Optison.

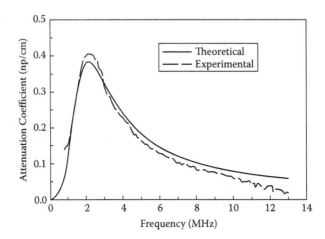

Figure 7.6 Experimental data and theoretical curve of attenuation coefficient as a function of frequency for Albunex with a mean diameter of 3.5 μm and a concentration of 8.8×10^4 microspheres/ml).

bubbles is lower than 1%, the mean scattering cross section of the bubbles, $<\sigma_s>$, can be calculated from

$$< \sigma_s > = \frac{\int_0^\infty \sigma_s(a, f)n(a)da}{N} \tag{7.11}$$

where $\sigma_s(a,f)$ is the scattering cross section of a bubble with a radius a at an ultrasound frequency f, N is the total number of bubbles, and $n(a)da$ is the number of bubbles with a radius between a and $a + da$ (Morse and Ingard, 1968). Since in a distribution of bubbles attenuation is dominated by scattering, the mean attenuation coefficient can be found in the same way by replacing σ_s with α. The attenuation coefficient of Abunex as a function of frequency is shown in Figure 7.6, where the maximal attenuation or scattering is seen to occur at approximately 2 MHz.

7.2 Nonlinear interactions between ultrasound and bubbles

The nonlinear response of a spherical bubble to a time-varying pressure field in an incompressible fluid has been analyzed by many investigators, including Rayleigh (1917) and Plesset (1949). It can be obtained by solving the Rayleigh–Plesset equation below under the assumptions that (1) the motion of the bubble is symmetric, (2) the wavelength is much greater than the bubble radius, (3) the bubble contains vapor and gas, (4) there is no rectified diffusion, which means the active pumping of gas initially dissolved in the fluid surrounding the bubble into the bubble by the sound field, and (5) the bubble oscillates according to the gas law with the polytropic constant ψ. The derivation of this equation can be found in Leighton (1994).

$$\rho_w a\ddot{a} + \frac{3}{2}\rho_w \dot{a}^2 = P_g\left(\frac{a_0}{a}\right)^{3\psi} + P_v - P_0 - \frac{2\delta}{a} - \chi\omega\rho_w a\dot{a} - P_a\cos\omega t \quad (7.12)$$

where a is the bubble radius, a_0 is the initial bubble radius, ρ_w is the density of surrounding medium, P_g (initial internal pressure of the bubble) $= P_0 - P_v + 2\delta/a_0$, P_0 is the ambient pressure, P_v is the vapor pressure, δ is the surface tension, χ is the damping constant, and $P_a\cos\omega t$ is the incident pressure. For an air bubble in water, $P_v = 2.33 \cdot 10^4$ dynes/cm^2 and $P_0 = 1.013 \cdot 10^6$ dynes/cm^2 at 1 atm. For the polytropic exponent or constant of gas $\psi = b\gamma$, where b is given by Equation (7.4). For air, $\psi = \gamma$ under adiabatic conditions and $= 1$ under isothermal conditions. The values for ψ for different gases have been measured (Crum and Prosperetti, 1983). Under adiabatic conditions, $\Psi = 5/3$, $7/5$, and $4/3$ for monoatomic, diatomic, and triatomic gases, respectively.

7.3 Modified Rayleigh–Plesset equation for encapsulated gas bubbles

The Rayleigh–Plesset equation was modified by de Jong (1994) to take the shell into consideration, resulting from the internal frictional loss and the restoring force caused by shell stiffness:

$$\rho_w a\ddot{a} + \frac{3}{2}\rho_w \dot{a}^2 = P_g\left(\frac{a_0}{a}\right)^{3\psi} + P_v - P_0 - \frac{2\delta}{a} - \frac{S_{shell}}{4\pi}\left(\frac{1}{a_0} - \frac{1}{a}\right) - \chi_t\omega\rho_w a\dot{a} - P_a\cos\omega t$$

$$(7.13)$$

where χ_t is the modified damping constant that accounts for the additional damping caused by shell friction and S_{shell} is the shell elasticity parameter, assumed to be a constant $= 8 \cdot 10^3$ dynes/cm by de Jong (1994, 1996).

7.4 Solutions to Rayleigh–Plesset equation

It is very difficult to solve the Rayleigh–Plesset equation analytically, but the solution can be found numerically (de Jong, 1994). The numerical results on the change in radius and velocity of an air bubble of 1.7 μm

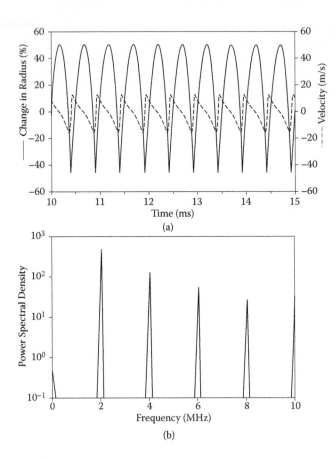

Figure 7.7 Response of an air bubble driven at its resonant frequency by an ultrasonic wave of 40 kPa. (a) Changes in radius and velocity of bubble wall, (b) corresponding power spectra.

radius in water at 20°C in the time and frequency domains, driven by a 30-cycle sinusoidal signal of 40 kPa amplitude at the bubble resonant frequency of 2 MHz, are shown in Figure 7.7. Initially, the bubble is assumed to be resting. Only the results for the last 10 cycles, a time when the system is assumed to have reached steady state, are shown. The bottom panel shows the spectra of the velocity waveforms. As expected, at either the maxima or minima of the radius variation of the bubble, the velocity is zero. Figure 7.8 shows the response for Albunex of 2.4 μm radius driven at 2 MHz, which exhibits a smaller swing in magnitude than a free bubble. Due to its larger stiffness, the radius of Albunex is larger to maintain the resonant frequency at 2 MHz. A value of 8000 dyne/cm was used for the shell elasticity S_{shell}. The additional damping due to shell friction was also included in the calculation (Chang and Shung, 1998).

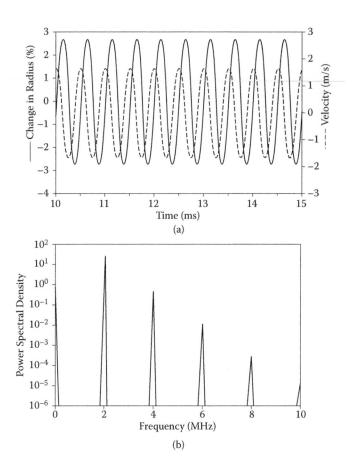

Figure 7.8 Response of Albunex driven at its resonant frequency by an ultrasonic wave of 40 kPa. (a) Changes in radius and velocity of bubble wall, (b) corresponding power spectra.

The computed scattering cross section of an air bubble of 1.7 μm radius and Albunex of 4.7 μm radius at first and second harmonics as a function of the driving frequency is given in Figure 7.9 (de Jong, 1994; Chang and Shung, 1998). The scattering cross section peaks for both first and second harmonics at 2 MHz. Beyond this frequency, it approaches the physical scattering cross section ($4\pi a^2$). Note that the second harmonic response is only prominent in the vicinity of the resonant frequency. For the air bubble there is also a prominent secondary maximum at half of the resonant frequency, which is a subharmonic frequency (not shown in the figure). The secondary maximum, however, is suppressed considerably for Albunex. Figure 7.10 shows the scattered power as a function of the radius from Albunex with a size

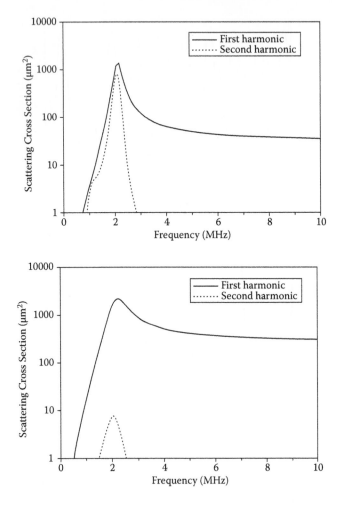

Figure 7.9 Calculated scattering cross section as a function of transmitted frequency at a driving peak pressure of 40 kPa. (a) For a free bubble of 1.7 μm radius (b) for Albunex of 2.4 μm radius.

distribution shown in Figure 7.3 for a transmitted frequency of 2 MHz and an amplitude of 40 kPa. The scattered power peaks at 4.7 μm for the first and second harmonic signals.

7.5 Harmonic imaging

An exciting new application of the gas-containing agents is found in harmonic imaging and Doppler measurements, where the effect of the surrounding structures on the image and results is minimized. Harmonic

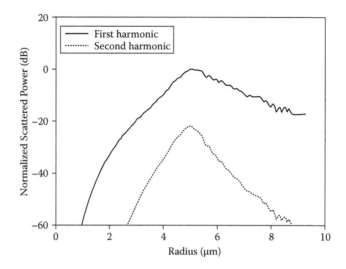

Figure 7.10 Normalized scattered power at the first and second harmonics as a function of Albunex radius. The size distribution shown in Figure 7.3 is used. The transmitted frequency and peak pressure are, respectively, 2 MHz and 40 kPa.

imaging or Doppler measurements following the injection of a gas-containing contrast agent are possible because only microbubbles resonate when impinged upon by ultrasound and emit ultrasound at harmonic frequencies. Ultrasound at harmonic frequencies will only be produced by anatomic structures that contain these agents. Tissues that do not contain gaseous contrast agents presumably will not produce harmonic signals. A good example is blood flowing in a blood vessel. Blood containing the contrast agent will produce harmonic signals, but the blood vessel will not. The contrast between the blood and the blood vessel will therefore be significantly improved in the resultant harmonic image if only the echoes at the harmonic frequency are detected by the transducer. The simplest approach that may be taken in harmonic imaging is to generate a wide-band signal acoustic signal. Only the harmonic signals are received for image formation, as illustrated in Figure 7.11. The array or transducer is excited with the first harmonic signal or fundamental frequency signal that can be achieved with a one-cycle sinusoidal signal, indicated by the thin solid line. The echoes received by the transducer are then filtered to collect the data only at the harmonic frequency indicated by the dashed line. The bold line indicates the original spectrum of the transducer. A major problem caused by such an approach is that it is impossible to completely remove echoes at the fundamental frequency due to spectral leakage, i.e., the overlapping area of the two spectra, thus corrupting the harmonic echoes. To overcome this problem, two other types of

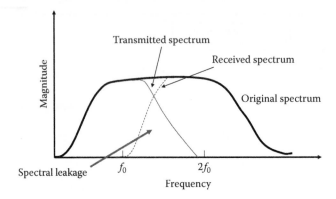

Figure 7.11 In harmonic imaging, the spectrum of a pulse within the bandwidth is divided into two bands, one for transmitting the pulse at fundamental frequency and one for receiving the second harmonic signal.

approaches have been used: pulse inversion and amplitude modulation (Averukiou, 2000), which are illustrated in Figures 7.12 and 7.13. In pulse inversion, two pulses of 180° out of phase are transmitted sequentially. The returned echoes are summed up. The echoes at the fundamental frequency will be canceled out, whereas those at the harmonic frequencies

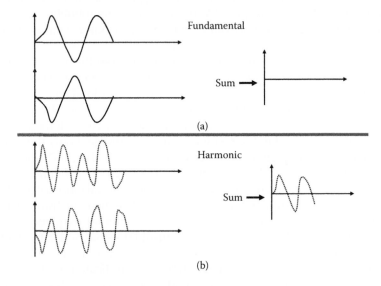

Figure 7.12 In pulse inversion harmonic imaging, two pulses 180° out of phase are transmitted. The returned echoes at fundamental frequency will cancel each other out upon summation (a), whereas the echoes at harmonic frequency will not (b).

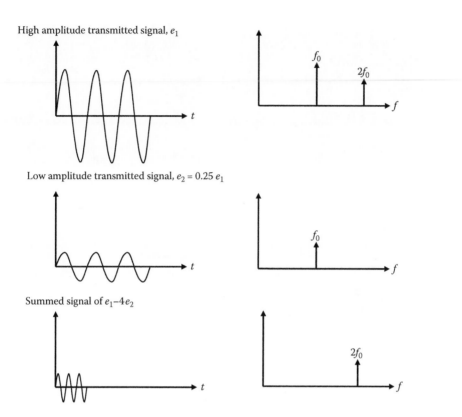

Figure 7.13 In amplitude modulation harmonic imaging, two pulses of different amplitudes, e_1 and $e_2 = 0.25\, e_1$, are transmitted. The larger pulse is assumed to produce a second harmonic signal, whereas the smaller one does not. Upon performing the mathematical operation $e_1 - 4e_2$, echoes at the fundamental frequency will be canceled out, whereas the echoes at harmonic frequency will not.

will not. In amplitude modulation, two pulses of different amplitudes are transmitted. The larger pulse will produce echoes at harmonic frequencies, but the smaller pulse will not. The signal at fundamental frequency may be subtracted out by adjusting the amplitude of the returned echoes. Only echoes at harmonic frequencies remain. Idealistically, these approaches are less affected by spectral leakage.

7.6 Native tissue harmonic imaging

Harmonic imaging can also be performed on tissues without the injection of a contrast agent. Harmonic signals are produced as the ultrasound pulse penetrates into the body because of the nonlinear interaction between the tissues and ultrasound energy, previously discussed in Section 2.8. Energy

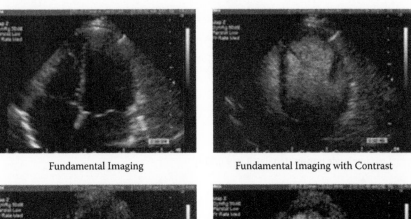

Fundamental Imaging	Fundamental Imaging with Contrast
Harmonic Imaging	Harmonic Imaging with Contrast

Figure 7.14 A four-chamber view of the heart with the interior of the cardiac chamber filled with bright echoes generated by a contrast agent. The borders of the cardiac chamber are better delineated in fundamental mode and harmonic mode. (Courtesy of Philips Ultrasound.)

at the fundamental frequency is partly absorbed, partly scattered, and partly converted into harmonic and subharmonic signals, which increase initially, reach a plateau, and then decrease. Similar approaches described in the preceding section can be used to perform native tissue harmonic imaging. Figure 7.14 shows a heart image at fundamental frequency and at the second harmonic with and without contrast.

Native tissue harmonic imaging has several advantages over conventional B-mode imaging. (1) It can penetrate deeper into tissues since more harmonic signals are generated until they are offset by the increased attenuation. Consequently, it is frequently observed that harmonic images are better when obese patients are imaged. (2) Harmonic imaging has better lateral resolution because the beam is narrower due to the higher receiving frequency. (3) Harmonic imaging is less noisy in the near field because harmonic signal is small in the near field. (4) Harmonic imaging has smaller side lobes. It also has the drawback that the higher attenuation shifts the center frequency of the harmonic signals to lower frequencies.

7.7 Subharmonic imaging

When gaseous contrast agents are excited by ultrasound at a frequency f, in addition to harmonic signals at $2f$, $3f$, etc., subharmonic signals at $f/2$, and ultraharmonics at $3f/2$, $5f/2$, etc., are generated as well (Shi and Forsberg, 2000). The advantages of subharmonic imaging are that (1) tissues do not appear to generate significant subharmonic signals and (2) attenuation of ultrasound energy at the subharmonic frequency is less. The disadvantage is that spatial resolution is poorer at $f/2$.

7.8 Clinical applications of contrast agents and harmonic imaging

When the contrast agents were first developed, their primary objective was in delineating cardiac structures. For instance, cardiac chamber borders can be better defined with the aid of a contrast agent, as illustrated in Figure 7.14. Since then, many applications have been found, including enhancing color Doppler flow images to better visualize smaller blood vessels, e.g., renal and hepatic arteries. The agent may be carried by the blood stream passively to an organ of interest, or it may actively seek out the targeted tissue by binding it with specific molecules that interact only with a certain group of molecules in a tissue, illustrated in Figure 7.15 (Lanza et al., 2000; Ferrara et al., 2007; Gessner and Dayton, 2010). The destruction of contrast agents by insonicating ultrasound has been used to measure blood flow stemming from the observation that the change in blood echogenicity following destruction is related to blood flow velocity, as illustrated in Figure 7.16. The most useful application of ultrasonic contrast agents appears to be in quantitating perfusion, that is, the blood supply to a certain region of an organ, which can seldom be done noninvasively. Figure 7.17 shows a color power Doppler image of a kidney following the injection of a contrast agent. The color portion indicates the region of the kidney with blood supply. Perfusion of a certain region in an organ may be quantified by measuring the wash-in and wash-out times and other parameters of the contrast agent from the change in echogenicity of

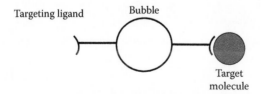

Conjugate bubble with a targeting ligand

Figure 7.15 A bubble conjugated with a ligand may target a molecule for binding.

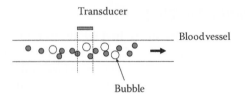

Figure 7.16 Blood flow velocity can be estimated by the rate of the increase in echogenicity of blood following the destruction of bubbles with ultrasound.

that region of tissue following the injection of a bolus of a contrast agent (Goldberg et al., 1994; de Jong, 1996). Its principle is identical to the indicator dilution method frequently used in medicine for estimating cardiac output. Figure 7.18 gives an example of quantifying perfusion with a contrast agent. The 80 refill time of a kidney tumor, which is the time needed to reach 80% of maximal echogenicity, estimated from the echo data following the injection of a contrast agent, is much lower than the surrounding structures. The magnitude of refill time is given by the color bar.

More recently, the interest in ultrasonic contrast agents has been focused on their potential in drug delivery. Drugs can be carried by these agents either in the interior or in the shell to a targeted organ where they are released. The releasing of a drug may be achieved by insonicating the agent with ultrasound. The agent may be carried by the blood stream

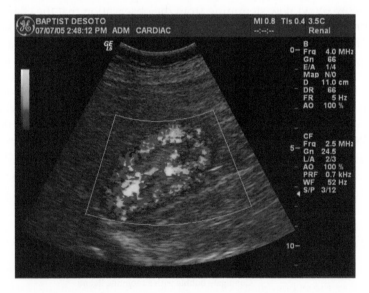

Figure 7.17 Color power Doppler of a kidney following the injection of a contrast agent. The perfused region is indicated by color. (Courtesy of GE.)

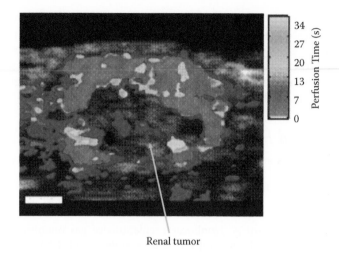

Perfusion Time (s)

Renal tumor

Figure 7.18 Refill time of a kidney estimated by quantifying echogenicity of the organ following the injection of a contrast agent. The center of the kidney has a tumor. Its refill time is very different from those of the surrounding structures. (Courtesy of Prof. Kathy Ferrara at University of California at Davis.)

passively to an organ of interest, or it may actively seek out the targeted tissue by binding it with specific molecules that interact only with a certain group of molecules in a tissue (Lanza et al., 2000; Ferrara et al., 2007). Figure 7.19 shows a sequence of optical images on the left acquired by a high-speed camera as a bubble bursts, maybe induced by insonification. The electron micrograph on the right shows a bubble with an oil shell that

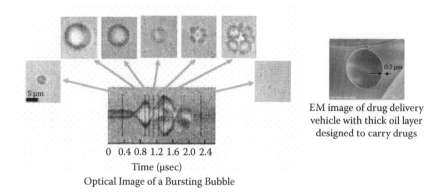

0 0.4 0.8 1.2 1.6 2.0 2.4
Time (μsec)
Optical Image of a Bursting Bubble

EM image of drug delivery vehicle with thick oil layer designed to carry drugs

Figure 7.19 Snapshots of the rupture of a bubble at different times, photographed by a high-speed camera. (Courtesy of Prof. Kathy Ferrara at University of California at Davis.)

can be loaded with a drug to be released upon ultrasound insonification. In this case, the bubbles are passively carried by the blood stream to the site of interest. The encapsulated bubble may also be conjugated with a targeting ligand, which targets a certain molecule on the endothelial surface so that the bubble actively seeks the molecule and binds with it (Figure 7.15). The drug that the bubble carries is then released upon insonification.

References and Further Reading Materials

Averukiou MA. Tissue harmonic imaging. *IEEE Ultrasonics Symp Proc* 2000; 2: 1563–1572.

Chang PP, Shung KK. Interaction of ultrasound with contrast agents. In Thomsen HH, Muller RN, and Mattery RF (eds.), *Trends in contrast agents*. Berlin: Springer, 1998.

Crum LA and Prosperetti A. Nonlinear oscillations of gas bubbles in liquids: An interpretation of some experimental results. *J Acoust Soc Am* 1983; 73: 121–127.

de Jong N. Improvements in ultrasound contrast agents. *Eng Med Biol Mag* 1996; 15: 72–82.

de Jong N, Cornet R, and Lancee CT. High harmonics of vibrating gas-filled microspheres. Part I. Simulations. *Ultrasonics* 1994; 32: 447–453.

Ferrara K, Pollard R, and Borden M. Ultrasound microbubble contrast agents: Fundamentals and application to gene and drug delivery. *Annu Rev Biomed Eng* 2007; 9: 415–447.

Gessner R and Dayton P. Advances in molecular imaging. *Mol Imaging* 2010; 9: 117–127.

Goldberg BB, Liu JB, and Forsberg F. Ultrasound contrast agents: A review. *Ultrasound Med Biol* 1994; 20: 319–333.

Lanza G, Hall C, Scott, M, Fuhrhop R, March J, and Wickline S. Molecular imaging with targeted ultrasound contrast agent. *IEEE Ultrasonics Symp Proc* 2000; 2: 1917–1926.

Leighton TG. *The acoustic bubble*. San Diego: Academic Press, 1994.

Medwin H. Counting bubbles acoustically: A review. *Ultrasonics* 1977; 15: 7–13.

Morse PM and Ingard KU. *Theoretical acoustics*. New York: McGraw Hill, 1968.

Plesset MS. The dynamics of cavitation bubbles. *J Appl Mech* 1949; 16: 277–282.

Rayleigh L. On the pressure developed in a liquid during the collapse of a spherical cavity. *Phil Mag* 1917; 34: 94–98.

Shi W and Forsberg F. Ultrasonic characterization of the nonlinear properties of contrast microbubbles. *Ultrasound Med Biol* 2000; 26: 93–104.

Wilson SR and Burns P. Microbubble-enhanced US in body imaging: What role? *Radiology* 2010; 257: 24–39.

chapter 8

Intracavity and high-frequency (HF) imaging

Conventional ultrasonic imaging systems typically use frequencies from 2 to 15 MHz. Scanners at lower frequencies have the advantage of a larger depth of penetration but suffer from poorer resolution. To improve spatial resolution, one obvious strategy would be to increase the frequency. The axial resolution is determined by the pulse duration or bandwidth of the pulse. For a fixed number of cycles per pulse, an increase in frequency would result in a reduction in wavelength and thus pulse duration. The relationship between frequency (wavelength) and lateral spatial resolution is given by Equation (3.29). These relationships are graphically illustrated in Figures 8.1 and 8.2. As ultrasound frequency is increased to 50 MHz, and an axial resolution and lateral resolution of better than 20 and 100 μm for an $f\#$ of 2.9 can be achieved, respectively. The price to be paid is an increase in attenuation. The effect of attenuation coefficient of a few types of tissues of clinical interest is shown in Figure 8.3. At 50 MHz, the depth of penetration for most tissues would be limited to 4–5 mm. Although, as was discussed, the depth of penetration may be increased slightly by introducing novel signal processing methods such as coded excitation, the range of frequencies that can be applied to a certain organ is limited.

8.1 Intracavity imaging

Intracavity imaging such as transesophageal, transrectal, and transvaginal imaging is a partial solution to achieving improvements in spatial resolution. Since imaging organs like the heart, prostate, and uterus/ovary from the body surface does not usually allow the utilization of frequencies higher than 5 MHz because they are deep-lying organs, probes may be modified to be inserted through open cavities of the body to be placed closer to these organs to allow higher frequencies to be used.

8.1.1 Transesophageal cardiac imaging

Phased arrays consisting of more than 48 elements at frequencies from 5 to 7.5 MHz can be mounted on the tip of an endoscope with a diameter

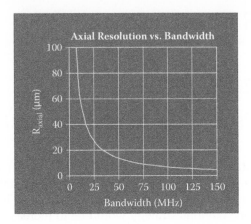

Figure 8.1 Calculated axial resolution as a function of bandwidth.

less than 10 mm for imaging the heart from the esophagus. The endo-scope allows the manipulation of the position and direction of the phased array. During scanning, the transesophageal probe is inserted into the esophagus and the tip is positioned against the wall of the esophagus under local anesthesia. A majority of the probes are capable of biplane imaging; i.e., two orthogonal images are produced. More advanced ver-sions can produce images in any direction by mechanically rotating the array. The most advanced probes have 2D arrays, allowing 3D imaging

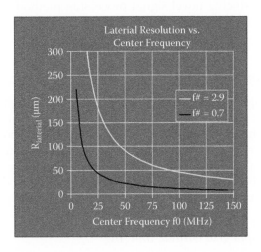

Figure 8.2 Calculated lateral resolution as a function of ultrasound center frequency.

At 50 MHz
$\alpha_{blood} \approx 2.5$ dB/mm
$\alpha_{cornea} \approx 1.1$ dB/mm
$\alpha_{iris} \approx 1.7$ dB/mm
$\alpha_{skin} \approx 10$ dB/mm

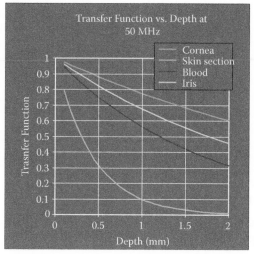

Figure 8.3 The effect of ultrasound attenuation of four different types of tissues plotted as a function of depth at 50 MHz. The transfer function is given by $e^{-\beta z}$, where β is the attenuation coefficient and z is the propagation depth.

of the heart in real time, which will be discussed in Chapter 8 in more detail. Transesophageal imaging of the heart yields better images of not only the whole heart because of the higher frequencies, but also the base of the heart, which cannot be adequately accessed by transthoracic imaging. An additional benefit is that transesophageal imaging allows continuous monitoring of the cardiac functions, which has proven valuable in anesthesiology during surgery. A photo of such a probe is shown in Figure 8.4. Commercial catheters (10 French units, 1 F = 0.33 mm outer diameter) mounted near the tip on the side of a linear array at a frequency of 8 MHz are also available for intracardiac imaging. The catheter can be guided to the heart with a guide wire via a peripheral artery.

8.1.2 Transrectal and transvaginal imaging

Probes at frequencies higher than 5 MHz are available for most imaging systems for insertion into the rectum or vagina for better imaging of the prostate and uterus/ovary. A linear array or curved linear array is mounted on the side or at the tip of a probe. A full bladder, which used to be recommended for transabdominal obstetrical imaging of a fetus, may now be replaced by transvaginal imaging. A photo of several transrectal and transvaginal probes is shown in Figure 8.5.

Flexible shaft

Enlarged view
of the tip

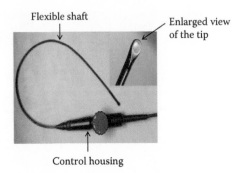

Control housing

Figure 8.4 A photo of a transesophageal probe. (Courtesy of Oldelft B.V., Delft, The Netherlands.)

8.1.3 Endoluminal imaging

Catheter-based imaging systems have also been used to image the gastrointestinal tract, including the colon, esophagus, and stomach (Liu and Goldberg, 1999). A few manufacturers have developed specialized ultrasonic imaging systems to accomplish the same by mounting ultrasonic transducers/arrays on the end of an endoscope. The frequency of the ultrasound probe ranges from 7 to 20 MHz, with a fluid-filled balloon at the tip. Linear arrays and radial arrays (elements mounted on the circumference of an endoscope) have been introduced recently.

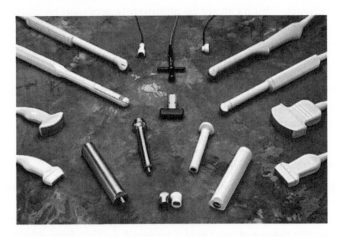

Figure 8.5 A photo showing several types of ultrasound probes, including linear arrays, linear curved arrays, Doppler probes, and transrectal and transvaginal probes (long and slender ones in the upper half of the photo). (Courtesy of Sound Technology, Inc., State College, PA.)

8.2 Intravascular imaging

Imaging of the wall of blood vessels for the purpose of estimation of the degree of stenosis and characterization of atherosclerotic plaques has been pursued for many years with a variety of imaging modalities (Pandian, 1989; Liu and Goldberg, 1999). X-ray angiography has been the gold standard in the past for assessing stenosis. The drawbacks of x-ray are that (1) it is a form of ionizing radiation involving the injection of a contrast agent, and (2) it is a 2D projection image of a 3D structure. More than two views are necessary to have a more accurate assessment of the stenotic vessel. As a result, its role is being challenged by both magnetic resonance imaging and ultrasound (Shung et al., 1992). Plaque composition characterization is of clinical importance in that it has been hypothesized that vulnerable plaques consisting of a lipid core with a fibrous cap are most likely to rupture, causing the formation of clots and serious clinical consequences, such as stroke and heart attack. Imaging options for characterizing plaque composition are quite limited. Fiberoptic angioscopy, in which an optic fiber is introduced via catheterization to the site of interest for the visualization of plaque surface, and transcutaneous ultrasound have been used. The former procedure, which involves injection of saline for flushing out light opaque blood, can only visualize the lesion surface, whereas the latter suffers from poor resolution. Intravascular ultrasound and optical coherent tomography (OCT) are possible alternatives to alleviate these problems (Liu and Goldberg, 1999; Bouma and Tearney, 2002). Intravascular ultrasound scanners typically are operated in the frequency range from 20 to 60 MHz, depending upon the imaging catheter used. There are two different types of imaging catheters on the market today. In one, a single-element transducer at a frequency from 30 to 60 MHz of 1.75 mm diameter, making an angle of 10° relative to the direction normal to the long axis of the catheter, is mounted near the tip of the catheter. The transducer is mechanically rotated at a very high speed (~1800 rpm) by a shaft. These catheters have a size of 3.5 to 6 F. In another, a 64-element array at 20 MHz having a 1.5λ pitch is mounted around the circumference of a 3.5 F catheter (1.2 mm outer diameter). The elevational width of the array is 0.7 mm. Also mounted on the catheter with the array are several integrated circuit chips that perform the functions of low-noise broadband preamplification and multiplexing. A synthetic imaging approach in which 1 element transmits and 14 elements receive is used to form the image. Figure 8.6 shows a catheter with a mechanically rotated transducer (top) and a catheter with an array wrapped around the circumference (bottom). The array catheter, although it has a higher frame rate, yields an image quality slightly inferior to that of the mechanically rotated type, primarily because of its lower frequency.

• **Mechanical Transducer**
  –Transducer that rotates on a drive shaft

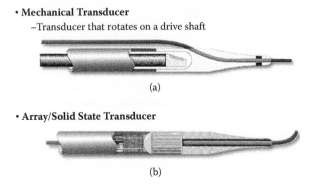

(a)

• **Array/Solid State Transducer**

(b)

Figure 8.6 (a) An intravascular imaging catheter with a mechanically rotated transducer. (b) A catheter with an array wrapped around the circumference. (Courtesy of Boston Scientific and Volcano Therapeutics.)

In addition to plaque characterization, intravascular ultrasound has been found to be useful in guiding the placement of a stent and monitoring stent restenosis. Figure 8.7 shows a 40 MHz image of an artery, whereas Figure 8.8 shows a 20 MHz image of a stent. At present, all intravascular ultrasonic imaging devices use side-looking catheters, which lack the capability of visualizing anatomic structures in front of the catheter. This capability is important in not causing any injury to the blood vessel itself, while being guided to the site of interest, such as perforation and dissection. Efforts are now underway in developing forward-looking

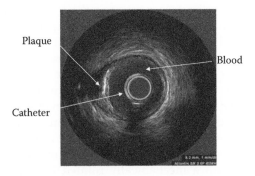

Plaque

Blood

Catheter

Figure 8.7 An image of an artery acquired at 40 MHz by a catheter with a rotating single-element transducer. (Courtesy of Boston Scientific.)

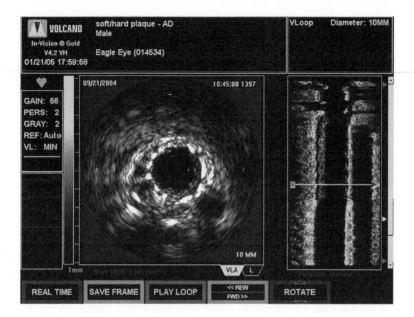

Figure 8.8 A 20 MHz imaging catheter is placed at the mid-stent level. The right panel shows a longitudinal view of the stent. The echogenic stent structure is clearly seen. (Courtesy of Volcano Therapeutics.)

intravascular catheters (Degertekin et al., 2006), and a forward-looking device that is a variation of the rotating single-element type is now commercially available.

A more recent trend in intravascular imaging is in combining two or more modalities taking advantage of the merits of each (Li et al., 2010). This will be discussed in more detail in Section 9.4.2.

8.3 High-frequency imaging

Scanners operated at frequencies higher than 20 MHz have been developed for applications in ophthalmology, dermatology, and small animal imaging. Typically these devices, called ultrasonic backscatter microscope or ultrasonic biomicroscope (UBM), obtain images by scanning a single-element ultrasonic transducer either in a sector format or linearly. The construction of a UBM is identical to that of a static B-mode scanner (Briggs and Arnold, 1996; Pavlin and Foster, 1995). Scanning can also be achieved by better utilizing the focus of the transducer by incrementally moving the transducer in the axial direction, called B-D (D stands for

Dimensions

• Pitch: 50 µm
• Elevation: 2 mm, self focused
  (f#=4)

Design Components

• Custom flex circuit
  interconnect
• 1 3 composite element
• Single matching layer
• λ/475 Ω coax for elect. imp.
  matching

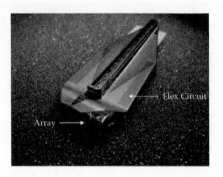

Figure 8.9 A 256-element HF 30 MHz linear array of one-wavelength pitch fabricated with conventional dicing technology.

depth) mode scan. A composite image is formed by combing the focused segments of multiple images acquired as the transducer is moved in the axial direction. This mode of scanning improves lateral resolution by sacrificing frame rate. Commercial UBMs can achieve a frame rate of 30 per second because the excursion range is extremely small. High-frequency scanners that utilize linear arrays have been commercially available for preclinical small imaging since 2009 (Foster et al., 2009). Extensive investigations are still being undertaken in developing HF arrays and associated imaging electronics (Ritter et al., 2002; Foster et al., 2009; Cannata et al., 2011; Hu et al., 2011) for preclinical and clinical applications. Conventional dicing technology may be used to fabricate linear arrays up to 50 MHz because dicing blades are only capable of dicing kerfs as small as 15 µm. For arrays of higher than 50 MHz, alternative technology such as micromachining, which will be discussed in Chapter 9, laser dicing (Foster et al., 2009), or deep reactive ion etching (DRIE) (Yuan et al., 2008) may have to be exploited. A 256-element HF 30 MHz linear array of one-wavelength pitch fabricated with conventional dicing technology is shown in Figure 8.9. The array with an aperture size of 2 × 6 mm had a bandwidth of 55% and a cross talk level of –27 dB. The design philosophy is similar to low-frequency arrays with one or more matching layers and a light backing. A laser- (excimer at 248 nm) diced 256-element 30 MHz array with a kerf width of 8 µm for a preclinical scanner (VEVO 2100) produced by Visualsonics (Toronto, Canada) is shown in Figure 8.10. The corresponding images obtained by this array, shown in Figure 8.11, clearly demonstrate the superior quality of the image, where all voids in the phantom are visualized, over that obtained with a UBM. This scanner is capable of performing conventional and color Doppler.

There are many clinical applications for high-frequency ultrasound. In ophthalmology, scanners at 20 MHz or slightly lower have been used

(a)

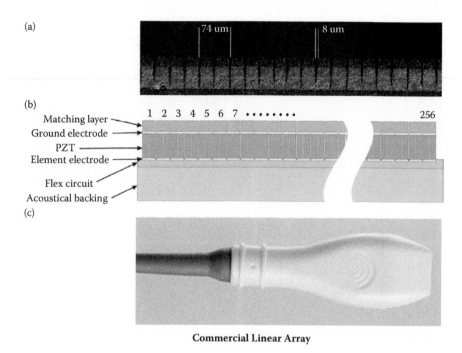

(b)

Matching layer
Ground electrode
PZT
Element electrode
Flex circuit
Acoustical backing

1 2 3 4 5 6 7 •••••••• 256

(c)

Commercial Linear Array

Figure 8.10 (a) A laser- (excimer at 248 nm) diced 256-element 30 MHz array with a kerf width of 8 µm for a preclinical scanner (VEVO 2100) produced by Visualsonics (Toronto, Canada), (b) the acoustic stack, and (c) photo array.

to interrogate the posterior components of the eye, including retina, whereas those at 40 MHz and higher are useful for visualizing the anterior segments of the eye, including cornea, for the purpose of monitoring the state of corneal transplant, and diagnosing tumors as well as glaucoma. Figure 8.12 shows the anterior segments of the eye obtained by a UBM at 50 MHz *in vitro*. The cornea, including the stroma, iris, and ciliary body, is clearly seen. Figure 8.13 shows an enlarged opening of the pupil when the light is turned off. Clinical applications of HF ultrasound in dermatology include characterization of tumors and assessing the size of structures in the skin, e.g., sebaceous gland. An image of the backhand skin obtained by a UBM at 50 MHz is shown in Figure 8.14. In ophthalmology and dermatology, HF ultrasound competes against OCT. The resolution of HF ultrasound is inferior, but the depth of penetration is superior.

Noninvasive imaging of small animals like mice and rats has recently generated a great deal of interest because, for gene and drug therapy, mice or rats are the preferred animal model. Due to their small size, clinical

Linear Array Image   **UBM Image**

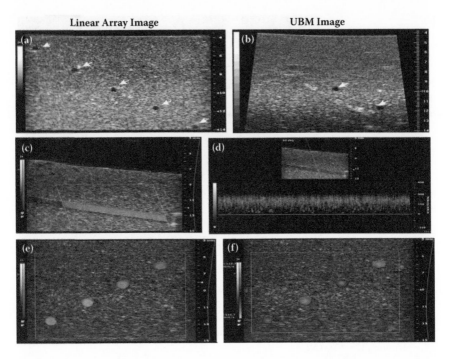

Figure 8.11 Images obtained by a 40 MHz linear array demonstrate superior quality to those obtained with a 40 MHz UBM. (a) and (b) Linear array and UBM images of cylindrical void phantom. Arrows indicate the locations of these voids. The UBM image is capable of only delineating voids near the focus of the single-element transducer whereas the linear array, because of its dynamic focusing capability, clearly discerns all voids. (c) and (e) Linear array color power Doppler images of a flow phantom containing cylindrical flow channels obtained on planes containing the flow channel and perpendicular to the channel. (d) Linear array duplex image with spectral Doppler obtained a pulsed Doppler. (f) Linear array color Doppler image showing direction of the flow in the phantom obtained by a 40 MHz linear array.

imaging devices are not capable of yielding sufficient resolution. MicroMR (magnetic resonance) and microPET (positron emission tomography) designed specifically for small animal imaging have been developed and are commercially available. The Visualsonics system is designed to specifically target this market. Figure 8.15 shows a 2D power Doppler image of a melanoma in an adult mouse obtained by such a scanner.

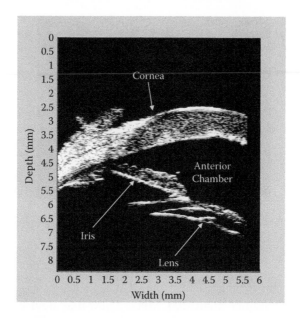

Figure 8.12 A UBM image of the anterior segment of the eye obtained *in vitro*.

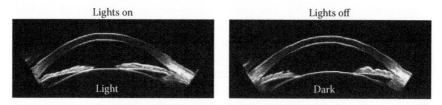

Ultrasound cross sections of the anterior segment of the eye

Figure 8.13 UBM images of the eye before and after turning off the light. (Courtesy of Artemis-2 VHF Arcscan (Ultralink).)

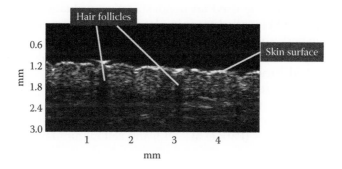

Figure 8.14 UBM image of human skin at 50 MHz.

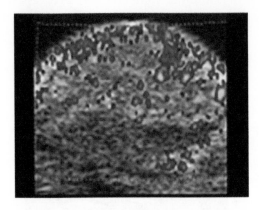

Figure 8.15 2D power Doppler image of a melanoma in an adult mouse. (Courtesy of Fuji Visual Sonics.)

8.4 *Acoustic microscopes*

At frequencies higher than 100 MHz, UBM-like devices have been developed for imaging cells and material structures. These devices are called scanning acoustic microscopes (SAMs) (Kessler and Yuhas, 1979; Briggs and Arnold, 1996). The construction is similar to that of a UBM with the exception that the transducer design is somewhat different. Conventionally, for fabricating transducers at these frequencies, a thin layer of zinc oxide is deposited on top of a tightly focused lens made of sapphire or quartz in order to minimize the effect of attenuation. More recently, thin-film piezoelectrics, e.g., PZT and PMN-PT, has been experimented with for developing transducers in this frequency range and results are promising (Zhou et al., 2011). Although a SAM at a few GHz has a resolution comparable to that of a light microscope, and the advantage of being able to penetrate light, opaque media has not gained acceptance in the biomedical community because of its limited capability and cost. It has been mainly used for nondestructive evaluation of materials. A variation of SAM is called scanning laser acoustic microscope (SLAM), in which the perturbation of the acoustic field generated by an ultrasonic transducer by an object is mapped by scanning a laser (Kessler and Yuhas, 1979; Briggs and Arnold, 1996).

Because of the recent interest in cellular bioengineering, ultrasound in this frequency range, i.e., ultra-high-frequency (UHF) ultrasound, has been exploited not only for imaging, but also for interrogating cellular mechanical properties (Park et al., 2012) and cell manipulation (Lee et al., 2011; Lee et al., 2012).

References and Further Reading Materials

Bouma BE and Tearney GJ. *Handbook of optical coherent tomography*. New York: Marcel Dekker, 2002.

Briggs A and Arnold W. *Advances in acosutic microscopy*. Vol 2. New York: Plenum Press, 1996.

Cannata J, Williams J, Zhang L, Hu CH, and Shung KK. A high frequency linear ultrasonic array utilizing an interdigitally bonded 2-2 piezo-composite. *IEEE Trans Ultrasonics Ferroelect Freq Cont* 2011; 58: 2202–2212.

Degertekin FL, Guldiken RO, and Karaman M. Annular-ring CMUT arrays for forward-looking IVUS: Transducer characterization and imaging. *IEEE Trans Ultrasonics Ferroelect Freq Cont* 2006; 53: 474–482.

Foster FS, Mehi J, Lukacs M, Hirson D, White C, Chaggares C, and Needles A. A new 15–50 MHz array-based micro-ultrasound scanner for preclinical imaging. *Ultrasound Med Biol* 2009; 35: 1700–1708.

Hu CH, Zhang L, Cannata JM, Yen J, and Shung KK. Development of a 64 channel ultrasonic high frequency linear array imaging system. *Ultrasonics* 2011; 51: 953–959.

Kessler LW and Yuhas DE. Acoustic microscopy. *IEEE Proc* 1979; 67: 526–535.

Lee CY, Lee JW, Kim HH, The SY, Lee A, Chung IY, Park J, and Shung KK. Microfluidic droplet sorting with a high frequency ultrasound beam. *Lab Chip* 2012; 12: 2736–2742.

Lee JW, Jakob A, Lemor R, and Shung KK. Targeted cell immobilization by microbeam ultrasound. *Biotechnol Bioeng* 2011; 108: 1643–1650.

Li X, Yin J, Hu CH, Zhou QF, Shung KK, and Chen ZP. High resolution coregistered intravascular imaging with integrated ultrasound and optical coherence tomography probe. *Appl Phys Lett* 2010; 97: 133702.

Liu JB and Goldberg BB. 2-D and 3-D endoluminal ultrasound: Vascular and non-vascular applications. *Ultrasonics Med Biol* 1999; 25: 159–174.

Pandian PG. Intravascular and intracardiac imaging: An old concept, now on the road to reality. *Circulation* 1989; 88: 1091–1094.

Park J, Lee JW, Lau ST, Lee CY, Huang Y, Lien CL, and Shung KK. Acoustic radiation force impulse (ARFI) imaging of zebrafish embryo by high frequency coded excitation sequence. *Ann Biomed Eng* 2012; 40: 907–915.

Pavlin CJ and Foster FS. *Ultrasound biomicroscopy of the eye*. New York: Springer-Verlag, 1995.

Ritter TA, Shrout TR, Tutwiler R, and Shung KK. A 30 MHz piezo-composite ultrasound array for medical imaging applications. *IEEE Trans Ultrasonics Ferroelect Freq Cont* 2002; 49: 217–230.

Shung KK, Smith MB, and Tsui B. *Principles of medical imaging*. San Diego: Academic Press, 1992.

Yuan J, Rhee S, and Jiang XN. 60 MHz PMN-PT based 1-3 composite transducer for IVUS imaging. *IEEE Ultrasonics Symp Proc* 2008; 682–685.

Zhou QF, Lau S, Wu DW, and Shung KK. Piezoelectric films for high frequency ultrasonic transducers in biomedical applications. *Progr Mater Sci* 2011; 56: 139–174.

chapter nine

Multidimensional imaging and recent developments

A majority of conventional ultrasonic imaging systems are equipped with a variety of probes, including linear arrays of different frequencies, phased arrays, and Doppler transducers, for performing required imaging functions and measurements. Despite that numerous improvements have been made in sharpening the image and eliminating artifacts, problems caused by a lack of focusing on the elevational plane or control of slice thickness remain. One glaring example is the degradation of image contrast outside of elevational focus. In order to alleviate this problem, 2D array is the ultimate solution (Light et al., 1998; Smith et al., 2002). Unfortunately, for a 128-element by 128-element 2D array, the electronic channel and cable count would be enormously large, expansive, and very difficult, if not impossible, to manage. As an intermediate step, multidimensional arrays such as 1.25D, 1.5D, and 1.75D have been developed to partially solve the slice thickness problem. One central issue encountered in all multiple dimensional arrays is that more time is needed for data acquisition and signal processing. Current scanners almost exclusively take the approach in which a pulse is transmitted only after all the echoes within the field of view have been received. To gain additional time without sacrificing image quality, the capability of parallel processing is essential.

9.1 Parallel processing

Parallel processing may be achieved by transmitting multiple pulses at the same time, as shown in Figure 9.1. An image of the liver obtained by such a commercial scanner is shown in Figure 9.2. This strategy, however, would make the scanners more expansive and electronics more complicated. A simpler and more cost-effective solution, shown in Figure 9.3, which used a linear array as an example, was proposed by Shattuck et al. (1984). A broader beam than that normally used in a linear array is transmitted, and the returned echoes are detected in 4 to 16 directions simultaneously, achieved by appropriately adjusting the time delays. In the initial approach (Shattuck et al., 1984), analog delays were employed. For reception at an angle of $\theta + \Delta\theta_i$, where θ is the angle of the transmitted broad beam and $\Delta\theta_i$ is the angle between θ and the ith received beam ($i = 1, ..., M$),

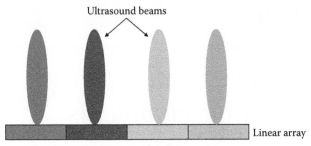

Four beams are transmitted at the same time

Figure 9.1 Parallel processing can be achieved by firing multiple beams at the same time.

depending on the design, $M = 4$ to 16, additional delay Δt_i can be applied to the original delay at a steering angle θ:

$$\Delta t_i = \Delta t_n(\theta, z_f) + \frac{ng}{c} \sin(\Delta\theta_i) \qquad (9.1)$$

where z_f is the focal distance of the beam, Δt_n is the time delay needed to focus the beam at z_f (see Equation 3.34) at an angle θ for the nth element, g is the pitch, and c is the sound velocity in the surrounding medium. This expression is valid only if θ and $\Delta\theta_i$ are both <26°.

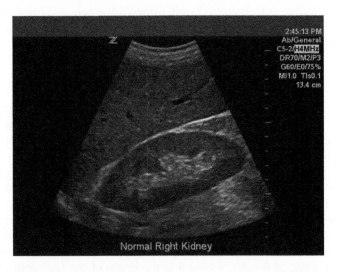

Figure 9.2 An image of liver obtained by a commercial scanner that uses the parallel processing scheme. (Courtesy of Zonare.)

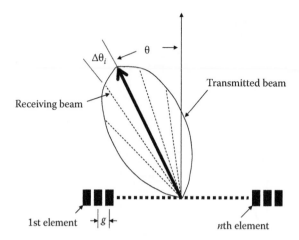

Figure 9.3 Parallel processing can also be achieved by sending a broader beam and receiving the returned echoes in multiple directions. θ denotes the steering angle. The receiving beams are much narrower than the transmitted beam.

For one transmitted pulse, four lines are received for $M = 4$. This means that the time needed to form one frame is reduced to one-fourth, representing an increase of frame rate by four times. The price to pay in achieving this is a slight degradation of lateral resolution in that the transmitted beam is broader and the electronics more complicated. Today, with faster electronics and computers, parallel processing is easily achievable digitally in a digital signal processing chip at a reasonable cost.

9.2 Multidimensional arrays

Multidimensional arrays have been classified into four categories: 1.25D, 1.5D, 1.75D, and 2D (Wildes et al., 1997), as illustrated in Figure 9.4, which shows only the side views of these arrays. A front view of a five-row 1.5D array can be found in Figure 3.40. For a 1D array the elevational aperture and lens focal distance are both fixed. For a 1.25D array, the aperture size is variable, but the lens focus is fixed. For near-field imaging, the switch is open and only the center row is used. For a 1.5D array, dynamic focusing is achieved by adjusting the delays of returned echoes or transmitted pulses just like what can be done on the azimuthal plane. Aperture apodization may also be implemented. A 1.75D array is similar to 1.5D, with the exception that there is no symmetry constraint. Typically, as in annular arrays, the areas of all rows may be made equal to ensure equal sensitivity and input electrical impedance, or a Fresnel pitch design may be implemented.

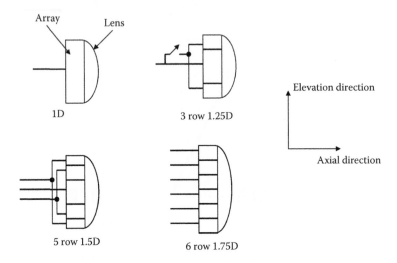

Figure 9.4 Side views of multiple dimensional arrays.

Only a full 2D array can allow dynamic focusing and beam steering in both azimuthal and elevational directions.

The major advantage that can be gained by going to multidimensional arrays is the better control of slice thickness and an improvement in contrast. The drawbacks are that (1) significant grating lobes are present in the elevational direction if there are too few rows of elements, (2) there is an increase in the footprint, (3) there are lateral resonances since the elevational width is reduced, (4) electrical impedance of the element increases since the element area becomes smaller, and (5) complexity in electronics increases.

A number of scanner manufacturers have developed 1.5D arrays. More than 1048 electronic channels (8 rows of 128 elements) are used for image acquisition. Significant improvement in image quality has been demonstrated.

9.2.1 2D arrays

To achieve 3D imaging in real time, a 2D array must be used. A 128-element by 128-element 2D array would allow the performance that can be achieved by a 128-element 1D array in the azimuthal direction to be extended to the elevational direction. 3D imaging by a 2D array may be accomplished in two ways: pyramidal scan and rectilinear scan, as illustrated in Figure 9.5 (Smith et al., 2002; Yen and Smith, 2002). In the former, the full 2D aperture is used for beam steering and focusing in both the azimuthal and elevational directions. In the latter, only a limited aperture is used, and the beam is moved linearly in a raster format to acquire the

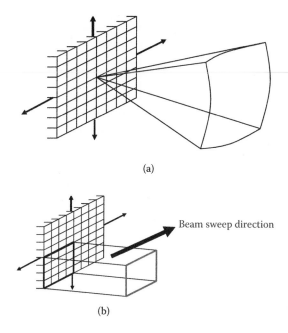

(a)

(b)

Figure 9.5 (a) Pyramidal scan by a 2D array. (b) Rectilinear scan by a 2D array.

full image in 3D. A rectilinear scan offers the advantage of reduced complexity, and thus cost, but suffers from an inferior resolution due to the smaller aperture size. Fabrication of the 128 × 128 2D array itself is not an unsolvable problem and can be done. The difficulty lies in the electrical impedance mismatch due to the small element size, the enormous amount of electronic channels if all elements are connected, and interconnection. Electrical impedance mismatch may be overcome with piezoelectric materials of high dielectric constant, multilayer piezoelectric materials that are acoustically in series but electrically in parallel (Goldberg and Smith, 1994), shown in Figure 9.6, or electrical impedance matching. Multilayer piezoelectric materials result in a reduction of $1/N^2$ in output electrical impedance of the array element, where N is the number of layers, recalling that the electrical behavior of a piezoelectric transducer is much like a capacitor near resonance. Figure 9.6 shows a capacitor of thickness L and area A. For an N-layer capacitor shown on the right, thickness reduces to L/N. The capacitance of this N-layer capacitor C_N becomes

$$C_N = N \frac{KA}{\frac{L}{N}} = N^2 C$$

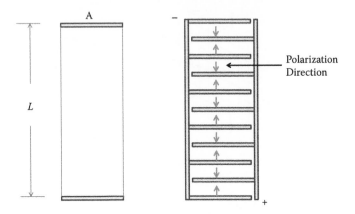

Figure 9.6 Multilayer piezoelectric materials.

where K is the dielectric constant and $C = KA/L$ is the original capacitance. Goldberg and Smith (1994) showed that for a 1.5D array element of $0.37 \times 3.5 \times 0.66$ mm consisting of three piezoelectric layers at 2.25 MHz of a prototype array, with a 2.5 pF cable shunt capacitance, a light epoxy backing and a $\lambda/4$ matching layer, a 100 Ω input electrical impedance, and a 197 pF clamped capacitance, were measured in comparison to an impedance of 800 Ω and clamped capacitance of 24 pF of a $0.37 \times 3.5 \times 0.77$ mm element consisting of a single piezoelectric layer of a control array of similar construction. An increase of 10 dB in round-trip sensitivity was observed from pulse-echo measurements. Multilayered piezocomposites have also been incorporated into array transducer design and shown to enhance their performances as well (Zipparo et al., 1999).

Multilayer flex circuits may be used to overcome the interconnection problem, but the cable size would still be unmanageable. A multilayer flex configuration for a 6×39 mm 1.5D array is shown in Figure 9.7, where (a) is a photo of the array assembly and (b) is an enlarged view of a section. The number of channel counts conceivably may be reduced by multiplexing or by adopting a sparse array approach (Smith et al., 2002; Lockwood et al., 1996). A fully sampled 2D array reported consisting of 9212 elements is now commercially available for 3D real-time volumetric imaging. It is not clear in this 2D array design whether there are equal numbers of elements in the azimuth and elevation. It is, however, known that for this 2D array, a subarray beamforming architecture is implemented. The elements first are grouped into 128 groups. Delays are applied to the elements in the group, summed, and cabled to the mainframe, where intergroup delays are applied and summed again. Presumably in this approach electronic channel count is reduced, but still allows a fast frame rate of 20–30 per second.

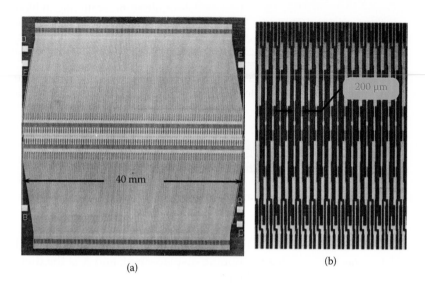

(a)   (b)

Figure 9.7 (a) A photo of a 1.5D array with multilayer flex. (b) Enlarged view of a section of the flex. The line width and via hole diameter are 25 and 50 μm, respectively. (Courtesy of D. Wildes, GE.)

Sparse arrays have been pursued for many years as an alternative to partially circumvent this problem.

A more recent advance in transducer technology that has a great potential in making the fabrication of a 2D array more cost-effective and in solving the interconnection problem is the capacitive micromachined ultrasonic transducer (cMUT) (Ladabaum et al., 1998; Oralkan et al., 2002; Mills, 2004). This approach differs completely from the traditional transducer design strategy and possesses the advantage in that semiconductor technology, which allows integration of transducers and electronics and miniaturization, is used. A cMUT cell is illustrated in Figure 9.8. The silicon nitride membrane and the silicon substrate form a capacitor, which makes the membrane vibrate upon the application of an AC voltage, V_{AC}, when biased by a DC voltage, V_{DC}. The gold layer is an electrode. The approximate dimensions of these structures are silicon nitride membrane 0.35–10 μm thick, the gap between the membrane and polysilicon $d_0 \approx 0.05$–12 μm, and silicon substrate ≈ 500 μm. Cell radius, a, goes from 10 to 200 μm. The force, F_c, acting on the membrane can be obtained from the following equation:

$$F_c = -\frac{d}{dx}\left(\frac{1}{2}CV^2\right) = -\frac{1}{2}V^2\left[\frac{d}{dx}\left(\frac{KA}{(d_0 - x)}\right)\right] = \frac{KAV^2}{2(d_0 - x)^2} \tag{9.1}$$

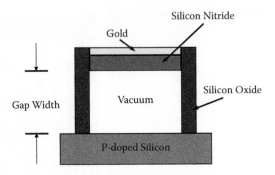

Figure 9.8 Construction of one capacitive micromachine's ultrasonic transducer (cMUT) cell.

where A is the area of the cMUT cell = πa^2, V is the voltage across the cMUT (a capacitor), x is the membrane displacement, and K is the dielectric constant. The static force when $V = V_{DC}$ and $x = 0$ is given by

$$F_{ST} = \frac{KAV_{DC}^2}{2d_0^2} \tag{9.2}$$

It is clear from this equation that the sensitivity of the device is inversely proportional to the gap width. It increases as the gap width decreases. It is also proportional to the bias DC voltage V_{DC}. The resonant frequency of the device is given by (Hietanen et al., 1992)

$$f_n = \frac{2.405}{2\pi a} \sqrt{\frac{\tau}{\rho_m}}$$

where τ and ρ_m are the tension and density of the membrane = 120 n/m and 3×10^{-3} kg/m^3 for silicon nitride. For $a = 5$ μm, f_n is about 12 MHz.

The cMUT element behavior has been analyzed with a simple first-order electromechanical model (Ladabaum et al., 1998), shown in Figure 9.9, where the medium in the cMUT is assumed to be a vacuum, and as a result, there is no mass loading effect. The force equation at the cell membrane can found by applying Newton's second law:

$$m\frac{d^2x(t)}{dt^2} - \frac{KAV(t)^2}{2(d_0 - x(t))^2} + kx(t) = 0 \tag{9.3}$$

where k and m are the mass and the spring constant of the membrane. This is a nonlinear second-order differential equation, which is very difficult to

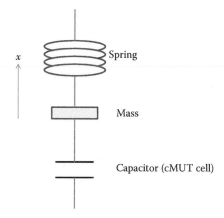

x

Spring

Mass

Capacitor (cMUT cell)

Figure 9.9 A first-order model of cMUT operation.

solve. To calculate the collapse voltage, set $V(t) = V_{DC}$ and assume no time variation; Equation (9.3) becomes

$$\frac{KAV_{DC}^2}{2(d_0 - x)^2} = kx$$

This third-order polynomial equation can be found to have a real root for $V_{DC} \gg kx$ at

$$x_{\text{collapse}} = \frac{d_0}{3}$$

and

$$V_{\text{collapse}} = \sqrt{\frac{8kd_0^3}{27KA}}$$

A reduction in spring constant k or a spring softening effect due to the electrostatic force acting on the membrane is often observed. The softened spring constant was found to be

$$k_{\text{soft}} = k - \frac{KAV_{DC}^2}{d_0^3}$$

As the resonant frequency of a spring-mass system is related to the square root of the spring constant, a drop in the resonant frequency of the cMUT is expected if the biased voltage is increased.

Another observation that can be made from the simple equation that relates the force acting on the capacitor and voltage, Equation (9.1), neglecting x, is that $F_c \approx V^2$. If an AC voltage is applied, $V = V_{DC} + V_{AC}$, it can be shown that

$$F_c \sim V_{DC}^2 + 2V_{DC}V_{AC} + V_{AC}^2$$

Assuming $V_{DC} \gg V_{AC}$, the time-varying part of $F_c \approx 2V_{DC}V_{AC}$. The larger the biased voltage, the greater the force or pressure that is produced.

Capacitive micromachined ultrasonic transducers (cMUTs), as the name implies, are fabricated utilizing MEMS methods. Two different approaches (Oralkan et al., 2002; Mills, 2004), surface machined and bulk machined, have been developed. The surface-machined approach developed by Ladabaum et al. (1998) is described in Figure 9.10. A clean P-type silicon wafer is prepared. A thin (1 μm) silicon oxide is grown on top of the wafer with a wet oxidation process as a sacrificial layer. In the next step, a layer of silicon nitride (0.35 μm thick) is deposited on top of the oxide layer via low-pressure chemical vapor deposition (LPCVD). A resist layer is then spin-coated. Electron beam lithography is subsequently performed, followed by plasma nitride and wet oxide etch. A second silicon nitride layer of 0.25 μm thickness is deposited on the released membranes. As the final step, a chrome and gold layer of 0.05 μm thickness is evaporated onto the nitride layer. A 3 MHz 128-element linear array was fabricated with cMUT (Oralkan et al., 2002). Each element of the array had a dimension of 200 × 600 μm consisting of 750 circular cMUT cells of 36 μm radius. Each had a silicon nitride membrane thickness of 0.9 μm and gap

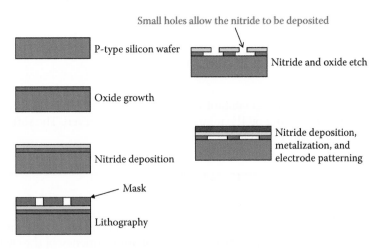

Figure 9.10 The MEMS process for cMUT fabrication.

MEMS structure on the surface; each cell has the width of a human hair

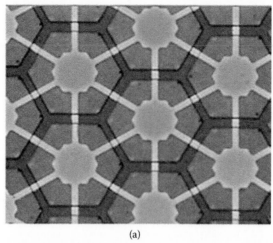

(a)

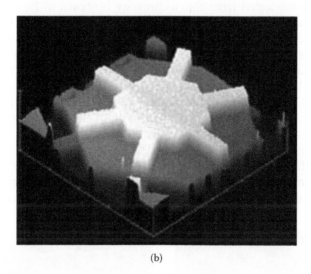

(b)

Figure 9.11 (a) Photo showing several cMUT cells. (b) Atomic force microscopic image of one cMUT cell. (Courtesy of Sensant Corp.)

width of 0.11 μm. The silicon substrate thickness was 500 μm. The device was found to have a bandwidth of 80% and a penetration depth of 21 cm in water. The level of cross talk was observed to be higher than that of comparable conventional linear arrays.

Figure 9.11(a) and (b) shows, respectively, a photo of several cMUT cells in which the lighter-colored structures are the cell membrane and conductive paths and an atomic force microscopic image of one cell. A 192-element

cMUT Linear Array

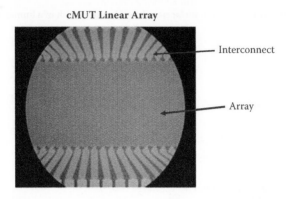

Figure 9.12 A photo of a cMUT 192-element linear array. (Courtesy of Sensant Corp.)

linear array fabricated from this technology is shown in Figure 9.12, and a corresponding image acquired by this array is shown in Figure 9.13, along with an image obtained by a conventional PZT array. An improved axial resolution is clearly seen due to the large bandwidth of cMUT. An additional advantage of cMUT is that the need for matching the acoustic impedance between the transducer and the loading medium is no longer necessary. There are, however, a few shortcomings with this technology: a slight decrease in sensitivity, much higher input electrical impedance, and the need for a bias voltage in the order of 100 V.

In another development, piezoelectric micromachined ultrasonic transducers (pMUTs) that use the bending mode of a piezoelectric layer spin-coated onto a silicon membrane have been studied for medical imaging as well (Dausch et al., 2008). This type of device makes use of the electromechanical

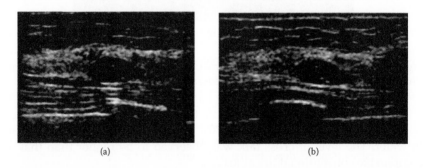

Figure 9.13 Image comparison of breast fibroadenoma at 9 MHz acquired by (a) a 192-element cMUT array and (b) a conventional PZT array. (Courtesy of Sensant Corp.)

coupling coefficient k_{31} of a piezoelectric material, i.e., displacement produced in the 1 direction upon the application of an electric field in the 3 polarization direction. It possesses the same advantage of cMUT in ease of fabrication and integration, with imaging electronics allowing the manufacturing of high-density arrays. An additional advantage is its larger capacitance than cMUT. The shortcoming is that k_{31} of a piezoelectric material is typically lower than k_{33}. A prototype 7.1 MHz 2D fabricated showed a –6 dB bandwidth of 57%. It should be noted that for pMUT, each pMUT cell represents an array element, unlike cMUT, where each array element is populated by many cMUT cells.

9.2.2 Sparse arrays

To reduce the number of elements and channel count, sparse arrays may be used. On a predetermined aperture, piezoelectric elements are randomly placed as shown in Figure 9.14, where all the elements may be used to transmit and receive, or some of the elements for transmission and some for reception. The advantage of a sparse array is countered by the decrease in sensitivity due to the reduction in aperture size and an increase in the side lobe pedestal or the noise floor outside of the main lobe. It has been shown to be proportional to 1/(number of elements) (Lockwood et al., 1996). To overcome this problem, a periodic sparse array has been suggested by Lockwood et al. (1996). The grating lobes caused by the large pitch in a sparse periodic array may be alleviated by selecting different pitches for the transmit and receive arrays. At a direction of φ_x shown in Figure 3.47 at a distance $r \gg L_a$, where L_a is the width of the array, the transmitted radiation pattern, as previously shown in Chapter 3, normalized with respect to the wavelength λ is given by

$$H_T(\delta) = \int a_T\left(\frac{x}{\lambda}\right) e^{jk\left(\frac{x}{\lambda}\right)\delta} d\frac{x}{\lambda} \qquad (9.2)$$

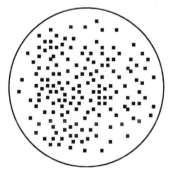

Figure 9.14 A random sparse array where the solid squares represent piezoelectric elements.

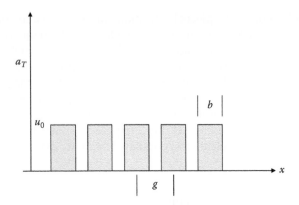

Figure 9.15 Transmit aperture function for a linear array of pitch g and element width b.

where $\delta = \sin \varphi_x$, λ is wavelength, k is the wave number, and a_T is the transmit aperture function. Again, this equation basically states that the radiation pattern of an aperture is the Fourier transform of the aperture function (Steinberg, 1976). For a linear array the aperture function can be represented by Figure 9.15, where b is the element width. If the acoustic independent variable chosen is medium velocity, $a_t(x/\lambda)$ is represented by a series of pulses with a medium velocity amplitude u_0. Here the distance x is normalized with respect to λ. If the receive radiation pattern is given by

$$H_R(\delta) = \int a_R\left(\frac{x}{\lambda}\right) e^{jk\left(\frac{x}{\lambda}\right)\delta} d\frac{x}{\lambda} \tag{9.3}$$

where a_R is the receive aperture function, the two-way pulse-echo radiation pattern would be

$$H_{TR}(\delta) = H_T(\delta)H_R(\delta) = FT[a_T]FT[a_T] = FT[a_T * a_R] \tag{9.4}$$

where * denotes convolution and $E(x/\lambda) = a_T(x/\lambda) \cdot aR(x/\lambda)$ is frequently called the effective aperture function or co-array function (Steinberg, 1976). In the far field of the array, i.e., $r \gg L$, the rectangular pulses may be represented by impulses, as shown in Figure 9.16. Assuming that there are N_T and N_R elements in the transmit and receive apertures, respectively, following the convolution, the number of elements in the effective aperture should be $N_{TR} = N_T + N_R - 1$ with a width of $2L$ and a pitch of ½λ. There are a variety of ways to reconstruct the effective aperture from the transmit and receive aperture functions. Figure 9.17 illustrates two of

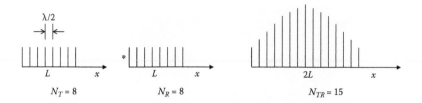

Figure 9.16 Desirable effective aperture function can be achieved by convoluting a transmit aperture function with a receive aperture function.

them (Lockwood et al., 1996). This approach is only valid for the far field of a nonfocused array and at the focus of a phased array. In addition, a combination of apodization and addition of extra elements is necessary to make it work successfully.

9.3 3D imaging

Three-dimensional ultrasound is an important new area of development. It exploits the tomographical capability of ultrasound by acquiring multiple slices of the images. 3D reconstruction can be accomplished offline or in real time using 2D arrays and parallel processing (Nelson, 2000). If a scanner is capable of displaying the volumetric images in real time, it is often called a 4D scanner. Offline 3D imaging is achieved by freehand scanning with electromagnetic position sensing or by mounting the probe on a mechanical translator whose position is encoded. The data acquired are displayed following image processing by optimized algorithms on a high-resolution monitor. Currently 3D ultrasound images are displayed

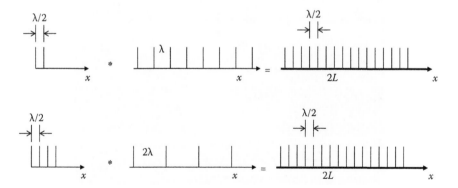

Figure 9.17 Two approaches that may be used to obtain a desired effective aperture function.

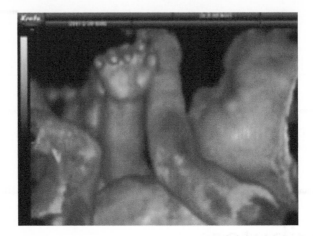

Figure 9.18 3D image of a fetus in uterus obtained offline. (Courtesy of GE Medical Systems.)

in two ways: a series of multiplanar images orthogonal to one another and rendered images that show the 3D structures. Rotation of the images is provided as an option. A 3D image of a fetus obtained offline and a 3D image of the heart obtained in real time or by a 4D scanner are shown, respectively, in Figures 9.18 and 9.19, where the gray-scale B-mode image represents heart anatomy and color image denotes blood flow.

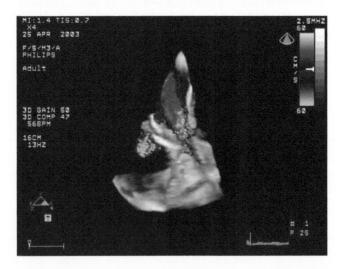

Figure 9.19 3D image of aortic valve in gray scale and the aortic regurgitant jet in color obtained in real time. (Courtesy of Philips Medical Systems.)

Some examples of clinical applications of 3D ultrasound are visualization of the coronal plane of a fetus, which is not possible with 2D ultrasound, measurement of organ volumes, including the heart, and guidance of interventional procedures, including needle biopsy of the prostate. Like several other imaging modalities, the clinical impact of 3D imaging is not yet firmly established and worth further investigation. It is, however, clear that for 3D ultrasound to have a major clinical impact, its performance must match that of 2D ultrasound in terms of image quality and interactivity.

9.4 Recent developments

9.4.1 Photoacoustic imaging

A new noninvasive imaging method resulting from the photoacoustic (PA) effect has recently generated intense interest. The PA effect arises from the absorbed energy in a medium from an incident light beam being transformed into heat, causing local medium expansion and contraction, and thus a pressure wave or acoustic wave, as illustrated in Figure 9.20. Similarly, acoustic waves can be generated by the absorption of electromagnetic radio frequency (RF) waves as well. This observation of sound generated by light was first reported in 1880 by Alexander Graham Bell.

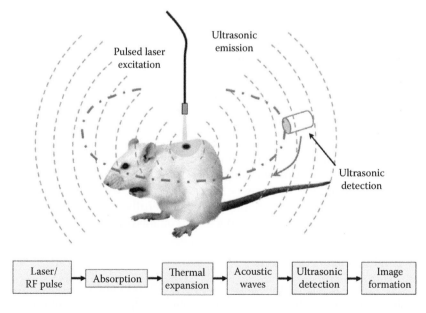

Figure 9.20 Principles of photoacoustic imaging. (Courtesy of Dr. LH Wang, Washington University.)

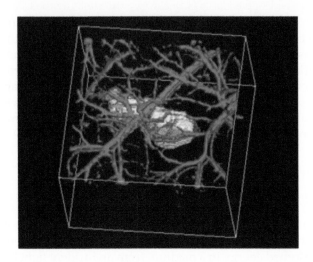

Figure 9.21 3D photoacoustic image of a melanoma surrounded by microvasculature in a mouse obtained *in vivo,* 584–764 nm light, 50 MHz ultrasonic transducer. (Courtesy of Dr. LH Wang, Washington University.)

The motto of PA imaging has been that it yields an image with optical contrast, but with ultrasound resolution, because the optical absorption characteristics of a medium determine the contrast of the image, while the receiving ultrasonic system determines the image spatial resolution (Wang, 2008). Photoacoustics is of particular interest in imaging microvasculature because the absorption of light in blood is much higher than in other tissues between 400 and 600 nm. Figure 9.21 shows a 3D photoacoustic image of a melanoma in a mouse obtained *in vivo* with a 584–764 nm laser and a 50 MHz ultrasonic transducer. The microvasculature surrounding the tumor in the background is clearly delineated. The anatomical structure imaged by PA in a body is determined by the light pulse duration, light wavelength, and ultrasound frequency and ultrasound bandwidth. Problems associated with PA imaging are (1) unknown optical attenuation in the propagation path of the laser beam and (2) unknown ultrasonic attenuation of acoustic signals between the source and the ultrasound detector. These factors must be carefully taken into consideration for PA imaging to evolve into a useful biomedical imaging tool.

9.4.2 Multimodality imaging

Much research is now ongoing in combining different imaging modalities to take advantage of the merits of each modality. Optical coherent tomography and PA offer better spatial resolution and contrast, respectively, than ultrasound, although ultrasound has a larger depth of penetration.

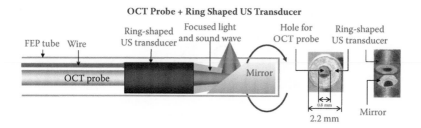

Figure 9.22 A hybrid OCT-ultrasound catheter-mounted probe.

Hybrid intravascular imaging combining ultrasound and optical coherent tomography and hybrid endoscopic imaging combining ultrasound and PA have been investigated (Li et al., 2010; Yang et al., 2012). Figure 9.22 shows a catheter probe of 2.2 mm diameter that combines ultrasound and OCT developed for intravascular imaging. In the center of the single-element transducer a hole is cut to allow the insertion of an optical fiber carrying light through it. Both light and ultrasound are reflected off a mirror to allow the collection of co-registered ultrasound and OCT images of blood vessel lumen as the catheter is rotated. The OCT, ultrasound at 35 MHz, and fused images of an excised human carotid artery obtained in a water tank are shown in Figure 9.23(a) to (c). In (c), the OCT image is given in color.

A hybrid endoscope for PA and ultrasound is shown in Figure 9.24. In this device, the mirror is rotated rather than the endoscope itself (Yang et al., 2012).

9.4.3 Portable scanners

Lightweight portable ultrasound scanners have found many medical applications because they can be readily used in emergency rooms and

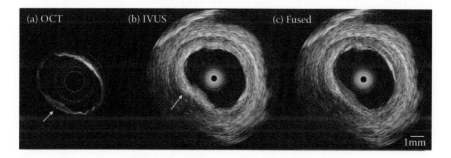

Figure 9.23 (a) OCT image. (b) Ultrasound image and (c) fused image of an excised human coronary artery obtained by the hybrid OCT-ultrasound probe *in vitro* in a water tank.

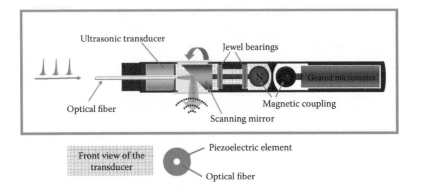

Figure 9.24 A hybrid PA-ultrasound endoscopic probe.

battlefields, and even in a physician's office if the physician has received proper training. As a result, scanners as small as an iPod have been developed and are commercially available. These scanners typically are operated at 3–5 MHz and equipped with a phased array capable of color Doppler. Figure 4.44 on pages 138 and 139 shows, respectively, two portable scanners and a pocket-sized scanner developed by three different manufacturers. The scanners shown in Figures 4.44(a) and (b) may weigh less than 11 pounds and have very few knobs, whereas the device in Figure 4.44(c) weighs only 390 g and has a 3.5 in. display with a sector angle of 75° and a depth of penetration of 24 cm at 3 MHz.

References and Further Reading Materials

Dausch DE, Castellucci JB, Chou DR, and von Ramm OT. Theory and operation of a 2-D array piezoelectric micromachined ultrasound transducer. *IEEE Trans Ultrasonics Ferroelect Freq Cont* 2008; 55: 2484–2492.

Goldberg RL and Smith SW. Multilayer piezoelectric ceramics for 2D array transducers. *IEEE Trans Ultrasonics Ferroelect Freq Cont* 1994; 41: 761–771.

Hietanen J, Stor-Pellinen J, and Luukkala M. A model for an electrostatic ultrasonic transducer with a grooved backplate. *IEEE Meas Sci Technol* 1992; 3: 1095–1097.

Ladabaum I, Jin X, Soh HT, Atalar A, and Khuri-Yakub BT. Surface micromachined capacitive ultrasonic transducers. *IEEE Trans Ultrasonics Ferroelect Freq Cont* 1998; 45: 678–690.

Li X, Yin J, Hu CH, Zhou QF, Shung KK, and Chen ZP. High resolution coregistered intravascular imaging with integrated ultrasound and optical coherence tomography probe. *Appl Phys Lett* 2010; 97: 133702.

Light ED, Davidson RE, Fiering JO, Hruschka PR, and Smith SW. Progress in two dimensional arrays for real-time volumetric imaging. *Ultrasonics Imag* 1998; 20: 1–15.

Lockwood GR, Li PC, O'Donnell M, and Foster FS. Optimizing the radiation pattern of sparse periodic linear arrays. *IEEE Trans Ultrasonics Ferroelect Freq Cont* 1996; 43: 7–14.

Mills DM. Medical imaging with micromachined ultrasonic (cMUT) arrays. *IEEE Ultrasonics Symp Proc* 2004; 384–390.

Nelson TR. Three-dimensional imaging. *Ultrasonics Med Biol* 2000; 26 (Suppl 1): S35–S38.

Oralkan O, Ergun AS, John JA, Karaman M, Demici U, Kaviani K, Lee TH, and Khuri-Yakub BT. Capacitive micromachined ultrasonic transducers: Next generations arrays for acoustic imaging? *IEEE Trans Ultrasonics Ferroelect Freq Cont* 2002; 49: 1596–1609.

Shattuck DP, Weinshenker MD, Smith SW, and von Ramm OT. Explososcan: A parallel processing technique for high speed ultrasonic imaging with linear phased arrays. *J Acoust Soc Am* 1984; 75:1273–1282.

Smith SW, Lee W, Light ED, Yen JT, Wolf P, and Idriss S. Two dimensional array for 3D imaging. *IEEE Ultrasonics Symp Proc* 2002; 1509–1517.

Steinberg BD. *Principles of aperture and array systems*. New York: Wiley, 1976.

Yang JM, Favazza C, Chen R, Yao J, Cai X, Maslov K, Zhou QF, Shung KK, and Wang LH. Simultaneous functional photoacoustic and ultrasonic endoscopy of internal organs *in vivo*. *Nature Med* 2012; 18: 1297–1302.

Yen JT and Smith SW. Real time rectilinear volumetric imaging. *IEEE Trans Ultrasonics Ferroelect Freq Cont* 2002; 49: 114–124.

Wang LH. Prospects of photoacoustic tomography. *Med Phys* 2008; 35: 5758–5767.

Wildes DG, Chiao RY, Daft CM, Rigby KW, Smith LS, and Thomenius KE. Elevation performance of 1.25D and 1.5D transducer arrays. *IEEE Trans Ultrasonics Ferroelect Freq Cont* 1997; 44: 1027–1035.

Zipparo MJ, Oakley C, and He AM. Multilayer ceramics and composites for ultrasonic imaging arrays. *IEEE Ultrasonics Symp* 1999; 947–952.

chapter ten

Biological effects of ultrasound

In earlier years, ultrasound propagation in biological tissues was assumed to be a linear phenomenon for the sake of simplicity since it was believed that the imparted power by a diagnostic instrument was so low that non-linear effects could be ignored. As the requirement for better sensitivity (signal-to-noise ratio) and image quality grew, both the peak and average intensity used in diagnostic instruments increased. At sufficiently high ultrasonic pressure levels and intensities, it is inevitable that nonlinear effects occur. So do new acoustic phenomena. Among the most important are heating, wave distortion, cavitation, radiation force, and streaming (NCRP, 1983; Hamilton and Blackstock, 1998). Table 10.1 lists typical acoustic output values for ultrasonic diagnostic instruments (AIUM, 1992a; Patton et al., 1994; Zagzebski, 1996).

10.1 Acoustic phenomena at high-intensity levels

10.1.1 Wave distortion

As the power level of the acoustic wave is increased, the sinusoidal pressure wave is distorted. This is because when a medium is compressed, the propagation velocity, inversely proportional to the compressibility and the density, increases. Thus, in regions of increased pressure, the propagation velocity is greater, causing the pressure peaks to catch up with the pressure troughs. When this occurs, the sinusoidal waveform begins to look like a sawtooth waveform and significant energy is transferred to higher harmonics of the wave, resulting in a higher absorption, as illustrated in Figure 2.20.

10.1.2 Heating

Ultrasound energy is attenuated as it propagates in a medium. In biological tissues, a major portion of the energy is absorbed and converted into heat. At low ultrasound intensity levels, the heat produced is rapidly diffused out, resulting in little change in local temperature. However, as the intensity is increased, temperature rises. Adverse biological effects may occur if the temperature is elevated to higher than 38.5°C (Barnett et al., 1994).

Table 10.1 Typical Acoustic Outputs of Diagnostic Ultrasonic Instruments

Operating mode	Peak pressure (MPa)	I_{SPTA} (mW/cm²)	I_{SPPA} (W/cm²)	Power (mW)
B-mode	1.68	18.7	174	18
M-mode	1.68	73	174	3.9
Pulsed Doppler	2.48	1140	288	30.7
Color flow	2.59	234	325	80.5

10.1.3 Cavitation

The term *cavitation* is used to describe the behavior of gas bubbles in ultrasonic fields. Two different types of cavitation may occur: transient (or inertia) and stable cavitation.

Transient cavitation describes the phenomenon in which microbubbles suddenly grow and collapse in a liquid medium. The physical process can be described as follows: Bubbles in a medium are greatly expanded when pressure decreases rapidly. The pressure increases one-half cycle later, causing bubbles to collapse and disappear. For a very large pressure swing the radius increases markedly, reaching a peak well past the pressure minimum, and as the pressure reaches a peak, the bubble collapses. The internal bubble pressure can become very high, up to 80,000 atm, with a temperature approaching 10,000 K. Such high temperatures can cause decomposition of water into chemically active acidic components, causing deleterious biological effects. A phenomenon called sonoluminescence, in which flashes of light with duration less than a few picoseconds are generated, may accompany the collapsing of the bubbles (Leighton, 1994).

Stable cavitation, on the other hand, describes a phenomenon in which the bubbles do not collapse, as just described. Under this circumstance, the behavior of such bubbles is quite stable and is known as stable cavitation. Stable cavitation is more likely to occur at lower ultrasound intensities.

Cavitation can be suppressed by degassing the liquid, increasing the viscosity of the surrounding medium, or increasing the static external pressure applied to the system. It takes a finite amount of time for the gas bubble to respond to the pressure change. Therefore, cavitation is a frequency-dependent phenomenon. If the ultrasound frequency is high enough, it should not occur.

10.1.4 Radiation force and streaming

As ultrasound propagates in a fluid, transfer of momentum to the medium via absorption causes acoustic streaming in the direction of the sound beam. If a discrete object is present in the ultrasound beam, a radiation force is exerted on the object as discussed in Chapter 2. As the object moves, streaming of the fluid near the object may occur. If the object is an air bubble, the oscillation of the bubble can also cause streaming of the fluid. Since acoustic streaming is related to absorption, nonlinear interaction between ultrasound and a medium may increase the acoustic streaming manyfold. Acoustic streaming could induce shear stress on interfaces that border the fluid and the object.

10.2 Ultrasound bioeffects

Ultrasound bioeffects have been classified into thermal effects or nonthermal effects, such as those caused by cavitation. However, in reality, on animal preparations these effects are usually difficult to separate. A large body of data has been accumulated over the years from both water tank studies and animal studies in an effort to establish whether diagnostic ultrasound produces biological effects.

10.2.1 Thermal effects

Results that delineate the relationship between temperature elevation and exposure duration needed to cause cell death are similar to those found for hyperthermia-induced fetal abnormalities. They can be generalized to the following equation (Barnett et al., 1994):

$$t = t_{43} R_a^{T-43} \tag{10.1}$$

where t_{43} is the exposure duration needed to produce bioeffects at 43°C, T is the temperature, t is the duration of exposure at T, and $R_a = 0.25$ for $T < 43$°C and 0.5 for $T > 43$°C.

A review of the literature shows that there have been no lethal effects observed for T below 41°C, and it can be assumed that exposures that elevate temperature up to 1.5°C do not cause defects of embryonic development.

10.2.2 Thermal index

A parameter that takes into consideration the attenuation of the tissues, beam profile, and tissue thermal properties was jointly proposed by the American Institute of Ultrasound in Medicine and the National Electrical Manufacturer Association to more objectively indicate the thermal effect of ultrasound so that the practitioners can use the ALARA (as low a power level as reasonably achievable) principle in patient scanning. This index is displayed voluntarily by the manufacturers on the scanner (AIUM/NEMA, 1992). For ultrasound propagating in soft tissues during scanning, the thermal index (TI) is given by

$$TI = \frac{W_0}{W_{deg}} \qquad (10.2)$$

where W_0 and W_{deg} are, respectively, the average emitted power of the source in water defined by the beam profile and the estimated power needed to raise the target tissue by 1°C based on tissue thermal models. To take tissue attenuation into account, W_0 in Equation (10.2) should be replaced by the derated power $W_{0.3}(z)$ at a distance z from the source, assuming a constant attenuation coefficient for all soft tissues of 0.3 dB/cm-MHz, which is 0.035 np/cm-MHz. Therefore,

$$W_{0.3}(z) = W_0 \cdot 10^{-0.03 f_c z} \qquad (10.3)$$

where f_c is the ultrasound center frequency. Equation (10.2) may be used to calculate TI for a scanning transducer with a relatively small aperture size in soft tissues since the power would be the highest at the face of the transducer, where $z = 0$.

$$TI = \frac{W_0}{(210/f_c)} \qquad (10.4)$$

where W_0 is in mW and f_c in MHz. For a $W_0 = 100$ mW at 3 MHz, TI = 1.4. TI for nonscan mode and Doppler mode may be different from that of the scan mode because of differences in transducer aperture and the thermal model. TI for ultrasound propagating in a medium containing bones is also different from that given by Equation (10.3) (AIUM/NEMA, 1992). AIUM/NEMA recommends that if a device cannot output a power level with a thermal index exceeding 1, it is not necessary to display the TI. However, if it can exceed a TI of 1, TI should be displayed when it exceeds 0.4 in 0.2 increments.

10.2.3 Mechanical effects and mechanical index

Cavitation and other nonthermal effects induced by ultrasound have been shown to cause cell lysis, change in cell permeability, and lung damage. Cavitation threshold is found to be related to the rarefactional peak pressure of an acoustic pulse that is the peak of the negative going pressure

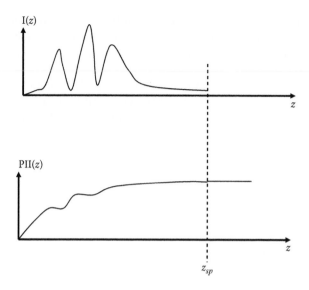

Figure 10.1 Definition of PII. The upper panel shows the pulse intensity as a function z. The bottom panel shows the spatial variation of PII.

(see, for instance, Figure 3.17), frequency, pulsing conditions, and properties of the propagating medium, including viscosity, gas content, surface tension, and temperature (AIUM/NEMA, 1992). Taking these parameters into consideration, the mechanical index (MI) is defined as

$$MI = \frac{p_{r0.3}(z_{sp})}{\sqrt{f_c}} \tag{10.5}$$

where $p_{r0.3}$ is the derated peak rarefactional pressure in MPa by 0.3 dB/cm-MHz, Z_{sp} is the axial distance where the derated pulse intensity integral $(PII_{0.3}) = \int I_{0.3}(z)$, and dz is maximal. PII is illustrated in Figure 10.1. Therefore, $I_{SPPA} = PII/\text{pulse duration}$. The maximal allowable MI is 1.9 equivalent to an $I_{SPPA0.3}$ of 190 W/cm².

Although MI has been adopted as a voluntary standard for assessing the mechanical bioeffects of ultrasound, it has several drawbacks. It does not consider (1) the dwell time, i.e., time involved in patient examination, (2) patient temperature, and (3) the effect of stable cavitation and other nonthermal mechanical effects. Further, MI was developed based on *in vitro* experiments using gas-containing polystyrene spheres.

Although the data that have been collected on bioeffects of ultrasound are frequently inconsistent and controversial, it is safe to conclude at the moment from extensive epidemiological studies and the body of data that is available in the literature (AIUM, 1992b) that in the low megahertz frequency range no adverse bioeffects have been observed on nonhuman biological tissues exposed *in vivo* under experimental ultrasound conditions if:

1. When a thermal mechanism is involved, these conditions are for unfocused beam I_{SPTA} below 100 mW/cm^2 and for focused beam I_{SPTA} below 1 W/cm^2, or thermal index below 2. Furthermore, adverse bioeffects have not been observed for higher values of TI when it is less than

$$6 - \frac{\log_{10} t}{0.6}$$

where t is the exposure time in minutes.

2. When a nonthermal mechanism is involved, these conditions are for in situ peak rarefactional pressure below approximately 0.3 MPa or MI < approximately 0.3 in tissues that contain well-defined gas bodies. Furthermore, no such adverse effects have been reported for other tissues.

In summary, the current consensus on possible bioeffects of ultrasound can be best illustrated by Figure 10.2, which shows that for long exposure time, as long as I_{SPTA} is below 100 mW/cm^2, no adverse bioeffects have been observed, and for short exposure time, the intensity allowable may be higher. As long as the energy imparted to the tissues is smaller than 50 joules/cm^2, no adverse bioeffects have been observed.

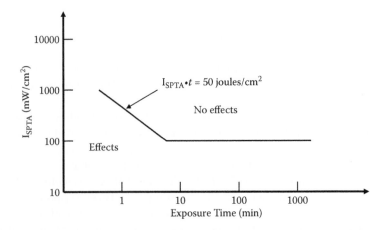

Figure 10.2 Graph summarizing the present knowledge of bioeffects of ultrasound.

10.2.4 Bioeffects associated with gaseous contrast agents

Gaseous contrast agents containing air or gas may act like stable nuclei for cavitation, and thus may pose an additional danger in ultrasonic imaging. Studies carried out on animals have found that microscale injuries to the renal and cardiac cells may occur, mainly caused by bubble rupturing when exposed to ultrasound. The threshold for bioeffects is much lower when there are bubbles and is inversely related to the square root of the frequency and peak rarefactional pressure, likely caused by cavitation. It was recommended that when a gaseous contrast agent is used, the MI of ultrasound energy generated by a scanner should be less than 0.4 (Miller et al., 2008).

The U.S. Food and Drug Administration (FDA) regulates the acoustic output from ultrasound scanners classified as class II types of devices. A 510K form has to be submitted prior to marketing and approved by the FDA. The most commonly used route for approval is one that is known as track 3. Devices must conform to an upper limit of *in situ* spatial peak intensity (I_{SPTA}) of 720 mW/cm^2, spatial peak pulse average intensity (I_{SPPA}) of 190 W/cm^2, MI of 1.9, and TI of 6.0. TI may exceed 6.0 provided that the level can be justified. Either MI or I_{SPPA} must conform to these limits. For ophthalmology, the poor vascularization of the eye leads to caution owing to the possibility of thermal effects, and lower limits have been set ($I_{SPTA} = 50$ mW/cm^2, MI = 0.23, TI = 1.0). For eye scanning, I_{SPPA} is not specified.

The output levels and bioeffect indices of a number of diagnostic ultrasound instruments have been reported by Patton et al. (1994). As a final note, bioeffects produced by ultrasound can also be used to its advantage for therapy, e.g., hyperthermia, high-intensity focused ultrasound (HIFU) surgery, drug delivery, and gene transfection (ter Haar, 2000; Miller, 2000).

References and Further Reading Materials

AIUM. *Acoustical output levels from diagnostic ultrasound equipment.* Laurel, MD: American Institute of Ultrasound in Medicine, 1992a.

AIUM. *Bioeffects and safety of diagnostic ultrasound.* Laurel, MD: American Institute of Ultrasound in Medicine, 1992b.

AIUM/NEMA. *Standard for real-time display of thermal and mechanical acoustic outputs indices on diagnostic ultrasound equipment.* Laurel, MD: American Institute of Ultrasound in Medicine, 1992.

Barnett SB, ter Haar GR, Zinskin MC, Nyborg WL, Maeda K, and Bang J. Current status of research on biophysical effects of ultrasound. *Ultrasonics Med Biol* 1994; 20: 205–218.

Hamilton MF and Blackstock DT. *Nonlinear acoustics.* San Diego: Academic Press, 1998.

Leighton TG. *The acoustic bubble.* London: Academic Press, 1994.

Miller DL, Averkiou MA, Brayman AA, Everbach EC, Holland CK, Wible J, and Wu J. Bioeffects considerations for diagnostic ultrasound contrast agents. *J Ultrasonics Med* 2008; 27: 611–632.

Miller MW. Gene transfection and drug delivery. *Ultrasonics Med Biol* 2000; 26: S59–S63.

NCRP. *Biological effects of ultrasound: Mechanisms and clinical implications*. Report 74. Bethesda, MD: National Council on Radiation Protection, 1983.

Patton CA, Harris GR, and Philips RA. Output levels and bioeffect indices from diagnostic ultrasound exposure data reported to FDA. *IEEE Trans Ultrasonics Ferroelect Freq Cont* 1994; 41: 353–359.

ter Haar G. Intervention and therapy. *Ultrasonics Med Biol* 2000; 26: S51–S54.

Zagzebski JA. *Essentials of ultrasound physics*. St. Louis, MO: Mosby, 1996.

chapter eleven

Methods for measuring speed, attenuation, absorption, and scattering

For a better interpretation of ultrasound images and an accurate measurement of the structure of a tissue, e.g., size or volume of a tumor, ultrasonic properties of biological tissues such as velocity, absorption, attenuation, and scattering must be known. There are a variety of methods that can be used *in vitro* to measure these properties. Performing these measurements *in vivo*, however, is a totally different matter as a number of methods developed to date have met with little success (Greenleaf, 1986; Shung and Thieme, 1993).

11.1 Velocity

11.1.1 In vitro *methods*

Ultrasound velocity can be measured either with a continuous-wave excitation or with a pulsed excitation (Schwan, 1969).

11.1.1.1 Interferometric method

This method, shown in Figure 11.1, uses continuous-wave excitation and has been used to measure the velocity in a liquid sample with negligible attenuation to an accuracy of 0.1%. A standing wave is set up between the reflector and the transducer. The wavelength can be determined by adjusting the position of the reflector. If the frequency is known, sound velocity can be easily calculated from Equation (2.2).

11.1.1.2 Pulse-echo method

The same arrangement in Figure 11.1 can also be used for pulsed excitation. A measurement of the time of flight $t = 2x/c$ of the pulse, where x is the distance between the reflector and the transducer would yield c. The accuracy of this method relies on the sharpness of the pulse and is affected by the attenuation of the sample, which can cause a change of the pulse shape. An improvement in accuracy can be made by substituting the sample with a liquid such as water, whose velocity is precisely known.

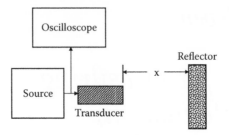

Figure 11.1 Experimental block diagram for *in vitro* ultrasound velocity measurements.

From measurements of two time of flights, t_s and t_r, in the sample and in the reference liquid, and the relationships

$$t_s = \frac{x}{c_s} \tag{11.1}$$

$$t_r = \frac{x}{c_r} \tag{11.2}$$

where c_s and c_r are, respectively, sound velocity in the sample and in the reference liquid, c_s can be found from the following equation:

$$\Delta t = t_s - t_r = x\left(\frac{1}{c_s} - \frac{1}{c_r}\right) \tag{11.3}$$

or

$$\frac{t_s}{t_r} = \frac{c_r}{c_s} \tag{11.4}$$

The advantage of using Equation (11.4) is that time-of-flight measurements are much more accurate than distance measurements. Since the distance measurement is eliminated by merely replacing the sample by a liquid of known velocity, this method is called the substitution method.

The pulse-echo approach can also be used to measure sound velocity in tissues. The problem is that it is often difficult to accurately estimate the thickness of the tissue. To maintain parallel interfaces between the transducer and the tissue, as well as between the tissue and the

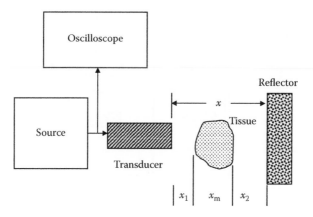

Figure 11.2 Experimental block diagram for *in vitro* ultrasound velocity measurements that eliminates the need for tissue thickness measurements by utilizing only time of flights.

reflector, the tissue must be compressed and an undesirable distortion of tissue structure may result. To alleviate this problem, a different approach, in which the need for measuring tissue thickness is eliminated (Kuo et al., 1990), may be used, as illustrated in Figure 11.2. Let us assume T_m and T_w are time of flights with the sample and without the sample in the propagation path, and t_1 and t_2 are time of flights for the pulse to travel from the transducer to the front and rear faces of the sample. Since

$$x_m = x - x_1 - x_2 = x - \frac{t_1 c_w}{2} - \frac{(T_m - t_2)c_w}{2} \tag{11.5}$$

$$\frac{T_w}{2} = \frac{x_1 + x_m + x_2}{c_w} \tag{11.6}$$

$$\frac{T_m}{2} = \frac{x_1 + x_2}{c_w} + \frac{x_m}{c_m} \tag{11.7}$$

where c_w and c_m are, respectively, sound velocity in water and in the sample. Substituting Equation (11.5) into Equation (11.7) and subtracting Equation (11.6) from Equation (11.7), it can be shown that

$$c_m = \left(\frac{T_w - T_m}{t_2 - t_1} + 1 \right) c_w \tag{11.8}$$

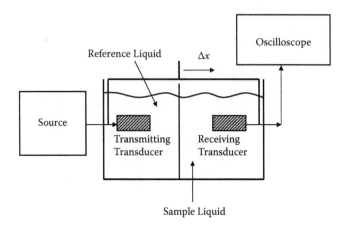

Figure 11.3 Experimental block diagram for the fixed path method for ultrasound velocity measurements.

This equation shows that the sound velocity in the sample can be determined from a measurement of four time of flights if c_w is known. An alternative to using a reflector to reflect back the transmitted pulse would be to replace the reflector with a hydrophone if the attenuation in the sample is high. In this way, the propagation path is reduced by half.

11.1.1.3 *Velocity difference method*
This method, which is extremely accurate (to 0.01%) for measuring sound velocity in a fluid, is shown in Figure 11.3. A reference liquid and the sample fluid are separated by a thin membrane. If a carriage carrying the transmitting and receiving transducers is moved by a distance Δx, it can be easily shown that the time of flight detected by the receiving transducer Δt is given by

$$\Delta t = \frac{\Delta x}{c_m} - \frac{\Delta x}{c_w} \tag{11.9}$$

All parameters in Equation (11.9) are known except for c_m. Continuous excitation can also be used with this method. Instead of measuring time of flight, the change in the phase angle is determined.

11.1.2 In vivo *methods*

Very few of the *in vitro* methods can be applied to *in vivo* conditions. As a result, a number of investigations on possible *in vivo* methodologies

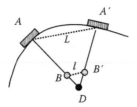

Figure 11.4 The image misregistration method for *in vivo* ultrasound velocity measurements in which a selected target is imaged at two locations.

have been attempted. One of those, called the image registration method (Chen et al., 1987), is shown in Figure 11.4. If a target tissue such as a blood vessel designated D can be found in the body by B-mode imaging, transducer A emits a pulse and target D will show up in the image as B, where $AB = c_0 \Delta t$, where c_0 is the assumed velocity and Δt is the time of flight. Similarly, for transducer A', $A'B' = c_0 \Delta t'$. For the triangle $AA'D$, it can be shown that

$$\frac{L}{l} = \frac{AD}{AB} = \frac{AD}{AD - AB} = \frac{AD}{AD\left(1 - \dfrac{c_0}{c_1}\right)} = \frac{1}{1 - \dfrac{c_0}{c_1}} = \frac{c_1}{c_1 - c_0} \tag{11.10}$$

where c_1 is the true velocity and $AB = (c_0/c_1)AD$. Equation (11.10) can be rearranged to obtain the following equation:

$$c_1 = c_0 \frac{L}{L - l} \tag{11.11}$$

which indicates that the true velocity can be estimated from the assumed velocity and the distances L and l. L can be physically measured and l estimated from the image. The true position of the target can be estimated by cross-correlation. Although this method appears to be promising, it has several problems, including the assumption that there is no refraction at tissue boundaries and the ability to find a target tissue. Using this method, Chen et al. (1987) found that *in vivo* sound speed in normal liver was 1.578×10^5 cm/s, whereas in nonfatty cirrhotic liver it was 1.547×10^5 cm/s.

An approach that uses a linear array is shown in Figure 11.5 and has been studied by Kondo et al. (1990). If the distance between two elements Δy and $\sin \theta_0$ is known and the propagation times along paths T_1AR_1, T_1BR_2, and T_2CR_2 represented, respectively, by t_{11}, t_{12}, and t_{21}, can be

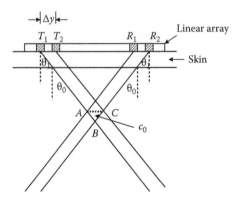

Figure 11.5 The crossbeam method for *in vivo* ultrasound velocity measurements in which a selected target is imaged by a linear array.

measured, c_0, the local sound speed in the volume of tissue defined by ABC is given by

$$c_0 = \frac{\Delta y}{\left(t_{11} - \dfrac{t_{12} + t_{21}}{2}\right) \sin \theta_0} \tag{11.12}$$

Here it is assumed that $\theta_0 = \theta_1$.

11.2 Attenuation

11.2.1 In vitro *methods*

Just as velocity measurements, there are a variety of methods that have been used for measuring the attenuation coefficient of biological tissues *in vitro*.

11.2.1.1 *Transmission methods*

Either narrowband bursts or broadband pulses may be used. The former yields better signal-to-noise ratio but can only be used to obtain the value at one frequency, whereas the latter allows the measurements of the attenuation coefficient over a frequency band but is susceptible to noise. These methods can be further classified as the fixed path method and the variable path method. As indicated by Equation (2.29), the pressure drops exponentially as the propagation distance increases. If the separation between a transmitting transducer and a receiving transducer is changed, a measurement of the change in the detected pressure should yield the attenuation coefficient if beam diffraction loss can be appropriately compensated. The advantage of the fixed path method over the variable path method is that there is no need to correct for beam diffraction. The fixed path method uses the same arrangement shown in Figure 11.3 for measuring ultrasound attenuation in fluids. Assuming that the attenuation coefficients in the reference liquid and the sample liquid are α_0 and α, and p_0 and p_1 are the pressures before and after the carriage movement, it is straightforward to show that

$$\alpha = \alpha_0 + \frac{1}{\Delta x}\ln\left(\frac{p_1}{p_0}\right) \tag{11.13}$$

This approach is not suitable for measurements on biological tissues. A substitution method has been developed to overcome this problem and is still the most reliable and most popular at present. An arrangement similar to that shown in Figure 11.2 is used. Since the detecting device must have a small aperture to minimize the phase cancellation effect or aperture averaging effect (Busse and Miller, 1981), typically in attenuation measurements a hydrophone is preferred as a receiver. This arrangement is depicted in Figure 11.6. The signals displayed on the oscilloscope received by the hydrophone without and with a specimen in the path, assuming that the scope has the capability of Fourier transform, as a function of frequency, are given by

$$V_a(f) = R_t(f)e^{-\alpha_0 x} \tag{11.14}$$

$$V_b(f) = R_t(f)e^{-\alpha_0 x}e^{-(\alpha-\alpha_0)x_m}T^2 \tag{11.15}$$

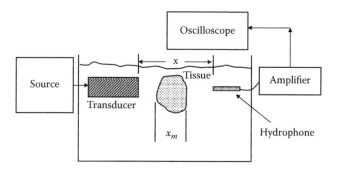

Figure 11.6 Experimental block diagram for *in vitro* ultrasound attenuation measurements.

where R_t is the transfer function of the experimental system, including the electronic and ultrasonic components, T is the acoustic transmission coefficient at the tissue-water interface, and α_0 and α are the attenuation coefficients in the reference liquid and the sample. Dividing Equation (11.14) by Equation (11.15),

$$\frac{V_a}{V_b} = e^{(\alpha-\alpha_0)x_m}T^{-2} \tag{11.16}$$

Since the transmission coefficient between a liquid and a soft tissue approaches 1, Equation (11.16) can be simplified to

$$\frac{V_a}{V_b} = e^{(\alpha-\alpha_0)x_m} \tag{11.17}$$

Equation (11.17) shows that the attenuation coefficient of the sample can be determined from a measurement of tissue specimen thickness x_m and the ratio of the detected signals if the attenuation coefficient of the reference liquid is known. The advantage of this method is that there is no need to know the experimental system transfer function $R_t(f)$. Unlike velocity measurements, the accuracy of thickness measurement is not as critical a factor in attenuation measurements. Specimen thickness, x_m, can be measured manually or with time-of-flight measurements.

11.2.1.2 Transient thermoelectric method

As was mentioned in Chapter 2, ultrasonic attenuation in tissues consists of two terms, absorption and scattering. Since in the medical ultrasound range, from 2.5 to 15 MHz, scattering loss is minimal, the transient thermoelectric method (Schwan, 1969; Parker, 1983) that measures absorption is also useful for measuring attenuation. In this method, a thermocouple is embedded in the volume of tissue of interest exposed by a rectangular acoustic pulse of known intensity; the temperature rise caused by the acoustic pulse measured by the thermocouple is shown in Figure 11.7. If

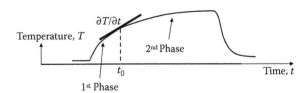

Figure 11.7 Temperature increase measured by a thermocouple after exposure to a pulse of ultrasound in a tissue.

the diameter of the thermocouple wire is sufficiently small, the approximately linear rise in temperature in the second phase is related to the absorption coefficient ~α by the following equation:

$$\alpha = \frac{C_p J}{2I}\left(\frac{\partial T}{\partial t}\right)_{t_0} \tag{11.18}$$

where C_p, J, and I are, respectively, the specific heat at constant pressure of the tissue, the mechanical-heat conversion factor (4.18 joule/cal), and acoustic intensity. $\left(\frac{\partial T}{\partial t}\right)_{t_0}$ denotes the slope of the temperature rise as a function of time at time = t_0. The first phase of temperature rise cannot be used because of the heat exchange occurring between the tissue and the wire. For this method to be valid, the wire diameter has to be small (<75 μm), the half-power beam width has to be greater than 3 mm, to minimize the heat loss by conduction to the surrounding regions, and the temperature rise < 1°. These guidelines restrict the application of the technique to high-frequency and tightly focused beams. A pulse decay technique where the viscous heating artifact is minimized has been developed to overcome these problems (Parker, 1983). In this method, a Gaussian intensity profile is assumed for the ultrasound beam (see Figure 2.8) and the beam is scanned across an embedded thermocouple of 51 μm diameter thermojunction, as shown in Figure 11.8. The intensity profile is assumed to be

$$I(x) = I_m e^{-\frac{x^2}{x_0}} \tag{11.19}$$

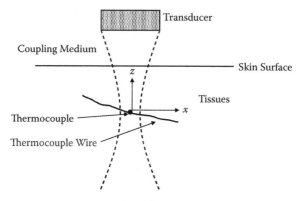

Figure 11.8 A transducer is scanned across a thermocouple embedded in a tissue.

where x_0 is a measure of the beam width. After an exposure of duration Δt and assuming no significant heat conduction during the duration, the temperature distribution along x should be

$$T(x) = T_m e^{-\frac{x^2}{x_0}} \tag{11.20}$$

where

$$T_m = \frac{2\alpha\Delta t}{C_p J} I_m \tag{11.21}$$

from Equation (11.18). The temperature decay at a point x at a function of time following exposure has been found theoretically (Parker, 1983) to be

$$T(x,t) = \frac{T_m}{4k_d t/x_0 + 1} e^{-\frac{x^2}{4k_d t + x_0}} \tag{11.22}$$

At $x = 0$ or on the beam axis,

$$T(0,t) = \frac{T_m}{4k_d t/x_0 + 1} \tag{11.23}$$

where k_d is the thermal diffusivity of the medium surrounding the heat sensor and equals 1.5×10^{-3} cm^2/s for soft tissues. Using Equation (11.23), T_m can be estimated from the time history of the temperature decay on the axis given x_0 estimated from Equation (11.19) following a measurement of the beam profile. Here it is assumed that the beam profile measured in a water bath is similar to that in tissues and not affected by attenuation. Then from Equation (11.21) the absorption coefficient β can be estimated since I_m, Δt, C_p, and J are all known. The advantage of this method over the transient thermoelectric method for highly focused beam was clearly demonstrated by Parker (1983).

11.2.2 In vivo *methods*

In vitro methods for attenuation measurements are difficult to be implemented *in vivo*. A few approaches have been studied for *in vivo* estimation of attenuation and can be classified into two categories: loss of amplitude methods and frequency shift methods (Greenleaf, 1986). The central idea for both is treating the tissue as a uniform distribution of

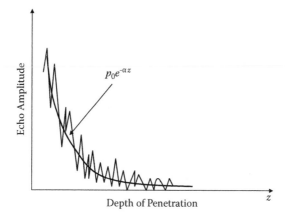

Figure 11.9 The echo amplitude scattered from a tissue decreases as a function of depth of penetration. The solid line denotes the fitted curve.

scatterers. If the difference in transducer beam characteristics at different depths in a tissue can be adequately compensated, the difference in echo amplitude from tissues at different depths of the same volume is related to the attenuation coefficient of the tissue and the separation in depth.

11.2.2.1 Loss of amplitude method
This method is illustrated in Figure 11.9, where the amplitude drop as a function of depth of penetration of the ultrasound beam or time of flight of the pulse is shown. If beam diffraction can be adequately compensated, the drop should be exponential and a curve fitting algorithm may be used to estimate the attenuation coefficient.

11.2.2.2 Frequency shift method
The frequency shift method can be accomplished either in the frequency domain by measuring the spectral difference or in the time domain by estimating the zero-crossing of the echo waveform, which was discussed in Chapter 5. This method is illustrated in Figure 11.10. Two regions, A and B, at different depths, of an A-line echo waveform are windowed for Fourier analysis, shown in Figure 11.10 (a) and (b). Various time window functions, e.g., Hamming, Blackman, and Henning windows, may be used to minimize spectral distortion. The two spectra are then divided to yield the slope of the attenuation curve shown in Figure 11.10(c) if beam diffraction can be adequately compensated. In logarithmic scale, the difference in the spectra yields the attenuation coefficient as a function of frequency. This process has to be repeated many times before any

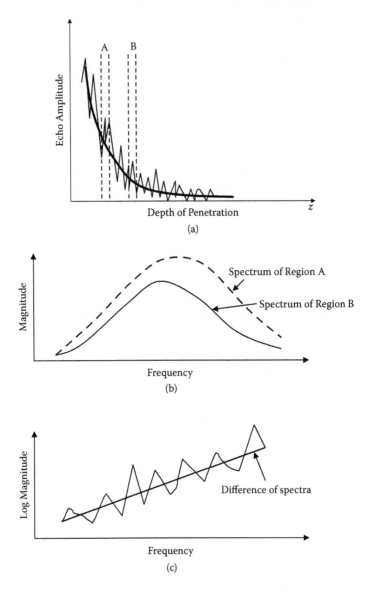

Figure 11.10 (a) The scattered echoes from two regions of a tissue, A and B, can be windowed for spectral or zero-crossing analysis. (b) Spectra of echoes from regions A and B. (c) The difference of the two spectra in log scale can be fitted with a line to estimate the attenuation coefficient.

meaningful results can be obtained because biological tissues are far from being homogeneous.

The shift in center frequency of the transmitted pulse can also be estimated from determining the zero-crossing of the echo waveform. Attenuation coefficients of normal liver and fatty liver with values from 0.45 to 0.5 dB/cm-MHz and from 0.6 to 0.8 dB/cm-MHz, respectively, have been reported from *in vivo* measurements on humans with these methods.

11.3 Scattering

The measurement of the scattering properties of tissues is of paramount importance because an ultrasonic image is formed from both specularly reflected echoes from tissue boundaries and diffusely scattered echoes from tissue parenchyma.

11.3.1 In vitro *methods*

The scattering properties of a medium can only be measured under two extreme cases: scatterer size >> wavelength and scatterer size << wavelength. As was discussed in Chapter 2, for a distribution of scatterers, only if the scatterer concentration n is very small is the intensity attenuation coefficient given by

$$2\alpha = n(\sigma_a + \sigma_s) \tag{11.24}$$

A measurement of the attenuation coefficient would yield σ_s, assuming $\sigma_s \gg \sigma_a$. This condition is satisfied only for large scatterers whose size is >> wavelength. Therefore, only under the case where the scatter concentration is extremely small and the scatterer size is >> wavelength can the scattering cross section be obtained from measuring the attenuation coefficient of the medium. Several methods, however, have been developed to measure the scattering properties of a medium for a distribution of small scatterers whose size is << wavelength (Shung and Thieme, 1993). The simplest is the narrowband substitution method, which was developed by Sigelmann and Reid (1973).

Suppose that a volume of tissue is insonified by an ultrasound beam as illustrated in Figure 11.11. Both the transducer and the tissue are immersed in saline solution in a water tank. The transducer is located a distance of R from the tissue and saline interface. Saline is preferred over water for a tissue sample to prevent permeation of water into the tissue. Here it is assumed further that R is >> transducer aperture and wavelength, so

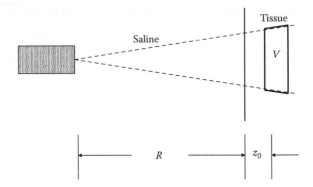

Figure 11.11 Experimental block diagram for *in vitro* ultrasound backscattering measurements.

that at $z > R$ the transducer can be treated as a point source. Under these conditions, the intensity of ultrasound beam at $R + z_0$ is

$$I(z) = \frac{P_0}{(R+z_0)^2} e^{-2\alpha_0 R - 2\alpha z_0} \tag{11.25}$$

where P_0 denotes the total power emitted by the transducer, the term $P_0/(R + z_0)^2$ is the spherical spreading of the energy emitted by a point source, α_0 is the attenuation coefficient in saline, and α is the attenuation coefficient in the tissue. If the transmitted ultrasound is a series of bursts at a frequency of f with a very narrow bandwidth, the intensity of the scattered wave from a region of tissue can be selected by time gating, which is illustrated in Figure 4.34 for measurement.

$$I_s(0) = \frac{I(z)\eta V}{(R+z_0)^2} e^{-2\alpha_0 R - 2\alpha z_0} \tag{11.26}$$

where V is the scattering volume, bounded by the beam width at $R + z_0$ and duration of the gate τ, = $Sc\tau/2$, c is the sound velocity in the tissue, S is the beam cross section at z_0, and η is the backscattering coefficient defined in Chapter 2. It should be noted that $\eta = n\sigma_b$, where σ_b is the backscattering cross section for very small n. However, for biological tissues, as was discussed in Chapter 2, σ_b is typically so small that it is impossible to measure. In order to alleviate this problem, the backscattering coefficient, which represents the intensity scattered into one solid angle in the backward direction per unit incident intensity with a unit of 1/cm-sr, is used. For this definition to be valid, the scattering from one unit of volume of scatterers must be so weak that there is no multiple scattering.

Otherwise, Equation (11.26) is not valid. Here it is assumed that individual scattering volumes are independent so as to allow the use of the product ηV to represent the total scattered intensity from a volume of V. The definition of scattering coefficient may be extended to dense distributions of smaller scatterers (Shung and Thieme, 1993), where scatterers are correlated. Biological tissues may be approximated as dense distributions of small scatterers because in the medical ultrasound frequency range the wavelength is typically much greater than the sizes of tissue components.

The power received by the transducer of aperture size A can be obtained by substituting Equation (11.25) into Equation (11.26), assuming $R \gg z_0$,

$$P_s = \frac{\eta A S \tau c P_0}{2R^4} e^{-4\alpha_0 R - 4\alpha z_0} \tag{11.27}$$

The backscattering coefficient can be estimated from Equation (11.27) by measuring S, P_0, α, and α_0 since all other parameters are known. The cross section of the beam S at the site of measurement may be measured precisely with a hydrophone or simply approximated by its –3 dB contour. The transmitted acoustic power P_0 is difficult to estimate because the transfer functions of the electronic and acoustic systems must be known. For practical purposes, the need for this knowledge is eliminated by performing an additional procedure that measures the reflected power from an ideal flat reflector at the position where scattering measurement is made. This is made possible by considering Figure 11.12, which shows a flat reflector is placed at a distance of R from the transducer, assuming $R + z_0 \sim R$. For a nonfocused transducer, it is possible to make the approximation that in the far field of the transducer, the transducer can be treated

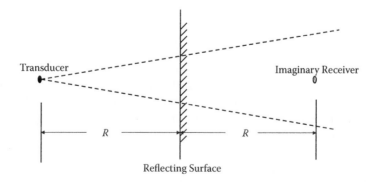

Figure 11.12 Diagram illustrating the mirror theory when a wave is impinging on a flat reflecting surface.

as a point source located at the center of the transducer aperture. Applying the mirror theory, the transducer as a receiver would appear as if it were located at a distance $2R$ from the source. The power received from the reflector by the transducer of aperture size A is then

$$P_r = \frac{A\Gamma P_0}{4R^2} e^{-4\alpha_0 R} \tag{11.28}$$

where Γ is the reflectivity of the reflector and approaches 1. Assuming $\Gamma \sim 1$ and dividing Equation (11.27) by Equation (11.28),

$$\frac{P_s}{P_r} = \frac{2Sc\eta\tau}{R^2} e^{-4\alpha z_0} \tag{11.29}$$

Rearranging this equation, it can be found that

$$\eta = \frac{R^2}{2Sc\tau} \frac{P_s}{P_r} e^{4\alpha z_0} \tag{11.30}$$

Equation (11.30) can be converted into dB scale by taking the log of both sides of the equation and multiplying by 10, that is,

$$10\log\eta = 10\log R^2 - 10\log(2Sc\tau) + (10\log P_s - 10\log P_r) - 10\log(e^{-4\alpha z_0}) \tag{11.31}$$

From this equation, it is easily seen that the backscattering coefficient, η, can be calculated by merely measuring the difference in the scattering power and reflected power in dB if all other terms are known.

This method has been used to measure the scattering properties of a number of tissues (Shung and Theiem, 1993). Results for several tissues are given in Table 2.1. As indicated earlier, the mirror theory is invoked to calculate the reflected power from a flat reflector. This approach is valid only for a nonfocused transducer. When a focused transducer is used, error will result (Yuan and Shung, 1986). The reason for this is illustrated in Figure 11.13, which shows that for a focused transducer, the imaginary point source is not located at R from the reflector. Not recognizing this crucial assumption in utilizing the substitution method has resulted in a large discrepancy in data reported in the literature for the backscattering coefficient of tissues.

A wideband pulse may be transmitted instead of a burst consisting of several cycles in scattering measurements. Following Fourier transform, the backscattering coefficient over a frequency band can be obtained by sacrificing the signal-to-noise ratio. A more accurate substitution method, that does not involve any approximation and is

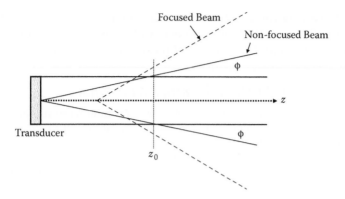

Figure 11.13 Only a nonfocused transducer can be approximated as a point source for far-field measurements. This approximation cannot be applied to focused transducers.

therefore much more computing intensive, was developed by Madsen et al. (1984).

For scattering measurements in highly absorptive media and at higher frequencies, a particulate reference medium whose scattering properties are well known may be used when the utilization of a focused transducer is necessary to achieve the required signal-to-noise ratio (Chen and Zagzebski, 1996; Wang and Shung, 1997).

11.3.2 In vivo *methods*

The gray level of a tissue in an ultrasonic B-mode image obtained by a scanner or the echogenicity of a tissue is related in a nonlinear manner to the ultrasonic backscattering coefficient of a tissue resulting from such signal processing steps as time-gain-compensation, echo amplitude to gray-scale mapping, etc., in a scanner. Only if these processing schemes can be adequately compensated, but it is extremely difficult to do, is there a one-to-one correspondence between echogenicity and the backscattering coefficient. By merely quantitating the gray level or echogencity of a tissue in video images acquired by a scanner *in vivo* following appropriate standardization procedures, a number of studies have shown that it is possible to differentiate diseased tissues from normal tissues in a variety of organs. More quantitative data can be retrieved by acquiring and analyzing radio frequency (RF) or raw data before signal processing, rather than the video data. In fact, there is a commercial system now that is equipped with an RF output for users who have need the RF data. Both backscattering coefficient and integrated backscatter (IB) have been measured from a number of tissues *in vivo* (Shung and Thieme, 1993). The most notable achievements have been made in the heart (Miller et al., 1985; Shung and Thieme, 1993) and the eye (Coleman and Lizzi, 1983; Shung and Thieme, 1993) for the purpose of tissue characterization.

References and Further Reading Materials

Busse LJ and Miller JG. Response characteristics of a finite aperture, phase insensitive ultrasonic receiver based upon the acoustoelectric effect. *J Acoust Soc Am* 1981; 70: 1370–1376.

Chen CF, Robinson DE, Wilson LS, Griffiths KA, Manoharan A, and Doust BD. Clinical sound speed measurement in liver and spleen in vivo. *Ultrasonics Imaging* 1987; 9: 221–235.

Chen JF and Zagzebski JA. Frequency dependence of backscatter coefficient versus volume fraction. *IEEE Trans Ultrasonics Ferroelect Freq Cont* 1996; 43: 345–353.

Coleman DJ and Lizzi FL. Computerized ultrasonic tissue characterization of ocular tumors. *Am J Ophthalmol* 1983; 96: 165–175.

Greenleaf JA. *Tissue characterization with ultrasound*. Boca Raton, FL: CRC Press, 1986.

Kondo M, Takamizawa K, Hirama M, Okazaki K, Inuma K, and Takehara Y. An evaluation of an in vivo local sound speed estimation technique by the cross beam method. *Ultrasonics Med Biol* 1990; 16: 65–72.

Kuo IY, Hete B, and Shung KK. A novel method for the measurement of acoustic speed. *J Acoust Soc Am* 1990; 88: 1679–1682.

Madsen EL, Insana MF, and Zagzebski JA. A method for data reduction for accurate determination of acoustic backscatter coefficients. *J Acoust Soc Am* 1984; 75: 913–923.

Miller JG, Perez JE, and Sobel BE. Ultrasonic characterization of myocardium. *Progr Cardiovasc Dis* 1985; 28: 85–110.

Parker KJ. The thermal pulse decay technique for measuring ultrasonic absorption coefficients. *J Acoust Soc Am* 1983; 74: 1356–1361.

Schwan HP. *Biological engineering*. New York: Wiley, 1969.

Shung KK and Thieme GA. *Ultrasonic scattering by biological tissues*. Boca Raton, FL: CRC Press, 1993.

Sigelmann RA and Reid JM. Analysis and measurement of ultrasound backscattering from an ensemble of scatterers excited by sinewave bursts. *J Acoust Soc Am* 1973; 53:1351–1355.

Wang SH and Shung KK. An approach for measuring ultrasonic backscattering from biological tissues with focused transducers. *IEEE Trans Biomed Eng* 1997; 44: 549–554.

Yuan YW and Shung KK. The effect of focusing on ultrasonic backscattering measurements. *Ultrasonics Imaging* 1986; 8: 212–219.

Index

Printed and bound by CPI Group (UK) Ltd, Croydon, CR0 4YY

22/10/2024

01777613-0008